METABOLIC CONFUSION DIET COOKBOOK FOR SENIORS

Unlocking the Power of Metabolic Confusion: Your Roadmap to Sustainable Weight Loss and Optimal Health

Stephen Kaiser

Table of Contents

INTRODUCTION

Welcome, dear reader, to the culinary adventure that lies within the pages of the "Metabolic Confusion Diet Cookbook for Seniors." If you've picked up this book, chances are you're on a quest for something more than just a collection of recipes – you're seeking a path to vibrant health, renewed energy, and perhaps a dash of culinary excitement along the way. Well, my friend, you've come to the right place!

Before we dive into the delicious details of this cookbook, let me extend a warm and heartfelt greeting. Whether you're a seasoned chef or someone who's just starting to explore the wonders of the kitchen, I want you to know that you're not alone on this journey. I understand that embarking on a new dietary plan, especially one as intriguingly named as the "Metabolic Confusion Diet," can feel like stepping into uncharted territory. But fear not! Together, we'll navigate these culinary waters with humor, empathy, and a generous sprinkling of delicious recipes to keep things interesting.

Now, you might be wondering, what exactly is this "Metabolic Confusion Diet" all about? It sounds like something straight out of a science fiction novel, doesn't it? Well, fear not, my curious reader, for I'm here to demystify the concept for you. At its core, the Metabolic Confusion Diet is not about deprivation or strict rules – it's about shaking things up, keeping your metabolism on its toes, and ultimately, finding a sustainable way to nourish your body and soul.

You see, as we age, our bodies undergo a myriad of changes – some welcome, others not so much. Our metabolism, once a fiery furnace that could digest just about anything we threw its way, begins to slow down, much like a tired old steam engine chugging up a hill. But fear not, my dear reader, for the Metabolic Confusion Diet is here to breathe new life into that weary metabolism of yours.

But enough about diets and metabolism – let's talk food! This cookbook is not just a collection of bland, uninspired recipes designed to keep you on the straight and narrow. Oh no, my friend, we're going to have some fun in the kitchen! From hearty breakfasts to satisfying lunches and delectable dinners, each recipe in this book is crafted with care and creativity, guaranteed to tantalize your taste buds and leave you feeling satisfied.

But before we jump headfirst into the culinary deep end, let's take a moment to acknowledge the elephant in the room – yes, I'm talking about the challenges that come with aging. We've all been there, my friend – the achy joints, the occasional forgetfulness, the uninvited gray hairs that seem to pop up overnight. But you know what? Aging may have its challenges, but it also brings wisdom, resilience, and a newfound appreciation for the simple pleasures in life – like a delicious meal shared with loved ones.

So, whether you're a sprightly senior with a passion for cooking or someone who's just looking to shake up their culinary routine, I invite you to join me on this culinary journey. Together, we'll explore the joys of cooking, the wonders of nutrition, and the endless possibilities that come with embracing a healthy, vibrant lifestyle. So grab your apron, sharpen your knives, and let's get cooking – because life is too short for bland food and boring diets

METABOLIC CONFUSION BASICS

Embarking on a new dietary journey can often feel like stepping into uncharted territory, especially when it comes to something as intriguingly named as the Metabolic Confusion Diet. But fear not, for in this chapter, we'll unravel the mysteries of metabolic confusion, explore its implications for senior health, and delve into the myriad benefits this approach holds for older adults.

Let's start by demystifying the concept of metabolic confusion. At its core, metabolic confusion is a dietary strategy designed to keep your metabolism guessing. Much like a savvy chess player constantly changing tactics to outsmart their opponent, metabolic confusion involves varying your caloric intake, macronutrient ratios, and meal timing to prevent your metabolism from becoming stagnant.

You see, our bodies are incredibly adaptable – they're like finely tuned machines that can adjust to changes in our environment. But over time, our metabolism can become accustomed to our eating habits, leading to plateaus in weight loss or metabolic slowdowns. That's where metabolic confusion comes into play. By introducing periodic changes to your diet, such as alternating between high and low-calorie days or varying your macronutrient distribution, you can keep your metabolism on its toes and maximize fat loss potential.

Now, you might be wondering, isn't this just another fad diet? And while it's true that metabolic confusion has gained popularity in recent years, especially within the realm of fitness and weight loss, it's important to approach it with caution and mindfulness. The key is to strike a balance between variation and consistency, ensuring that your dietary changes are sustainable and aligned with your long-term health goals.

How Metabolic Confusion Affects Senior Health

As we age, our bodies undergo a myriad of changes – some visible, others less so. Our metabolism, once a fiery furnace that could digest just about anything we threw its way, begins to slow down, much like a tired old steam engine chugging up a hill. But fear not, for metabolic confusion offers a ray of hope for seniors looking to revitalize their metabolism and reclaim their vitality.

One of the key ways in which metabolic confusion can benefit seniors is by preventing age-related metabolic slowdowns. By incorporating periodic changes to your diet, such as alternating between higher and lower-calorie days or varying your macronutrient distribution, you can help stave off the metabolic stagnation that often accompanies aging. This, in turn, can help support healthy weight management, enhance energy levels, and improve overall metabolic health.

But metabolic confusion isn't just about weight loss – it's also about optimizing nutrient intake and promoting overall well-being. As we age, our nutritional needs change, and it's important to ensure that we're getting the right balance of vitamins, minerals, and macronutrients to support healthy aging. By incorporating a variety of foods into your diet and periodically changing your eating patterns, you can help ensure that you're meeting your nutritional needs and supporting optimal health as you age.

Benefits of the Metabolic Confusion Diet for Seniors

So, what are the specific benefits of the Metabolic Confusion Diet for seniors? Well, for starters, this approach offers a flexible and customizable way to support healthy aging. Whether you're looking to lose weight, boost energy levels, or simply optimize your nutritional intake, metabolic confusion can be tailored to meet your individual needs and preferences.

Another key benefit of the Metabolic Confusion Diet for seniors is its potential to enhance metabolic flexibility. As we age, our bodies become less efficient at metabolizing nutrients, which can contribute to a host of health issues, including insulin resistance, inflammation, and metabolic syndrome. By periodically changing your eating patterns and introducing variation into your diet, you can help improve your body's ability to adapt to different fuel sources and support overall metabolic health.

Additionally, the Metabolic Confusion Diet offers a sustainable and enjoyable approach to healthy eating. Unlike traditional diets that rely on strict rules and rigid meal plans, metabolic confusion allows for flexibility and variety, making it easier to stick with over the long term. By incorporating a wide range of delicious and nutritious foods into your diet and experimenting with different eating patterns, you can keep your meals exciting and enjoyable while still reaping the benefits of metabolic confusion.

In summary, the Metabolic Confusion Diet holds great promise for seniors looking to optimize their health and vitality. By incorporating periodic changes to your diet, you can help revitalize your metabolism, support healthy aging, and enhance overall well-being. So why not give it a try? Your body will thank you for it

GETTING STARTED WITH THE METABOLIC CONFUSION DIET

Embarking on the journey of the Metabolic Confusion Diet marks a significant step towards reclaiming control over your health and well-being. In this chapter, we will delve into the essential aspects of initiating this dietary approach, from assessing your individual dietary needs to seeking guidance from healthcare professionals and crafting a personalized plan tailored to your unique requirements.

Assessing Your Dietary Needs

Before diving headfirst into any dietary regimen, it's crucial to take a step back and assess your current dietary habits, nutritional deficiencies, and health goals. Assessing your dietary needs provides the foundation upon which you can build a successful and sustainable Metabolic Confusion Diet plan.

Start by taking inventory of your typical eating patterns, including the types of foods you consume, portion sizes, and meal timing. Pay close attention to any dietary habits that may be contributing to weight gain, energy fluctuations, or other health concerns.

Next, consider your nutritional requirements based on factors such as age, gender, activity level, and any underlying health conditions. Are you getting enough essential nutrients such as vitamins, minerals, protein, and fiber? Are there specific dietary changes you need to make to address deficiencies or support optimal health?

Keep in mind that assessing your dietary needs is not just about counting calories or macros – it's about understanding how different foods impact your body and identifying areas for improvement. Consider keeping a food diary for a few days to track you're eating habits and gain insights into areas where adjustments may be needed.

Consultation with Healthcare Professionals

Once you have a clear understanding of your dietary needs and health goals, the next step is to seek guidance from healthcare professionals who can provide personalized recommendations and support. While embarking on a new dietary regimen can be empowering, it's essential to approach it with caution and seek professional advice to ensure it aligns with your overall health and well-being.

Schedule a consultation with your primary care physician or a registered dietitian to discuss your intentions to start the Metabolic Confusion Diet. Share your dietary assessment findings, health concerns, and goals for embarking on this journey. Your healthcare provider can offer valuable insights into how the Metabolic Confusion Diet may impact your specific health status and provide recommendations tailored to your needs.

During your consultation, be prepared to discuss any existing medical conditions, medications, or dietary restrictions that may influence your dietary choices. Your healthcare provider can help you navigate any potential challenges and provide guidance on how to safely implement the Metabolic Confusion Diet while addressing your unique health needs.

Creating a Personalized Plan

Armed with insights from your dietary assessment and guidance from healthcare professionals, it's time to craft a personalized Metabolic Confusion Diet plan that aligns with your goals and preferences. Creating a customized plan ensures that you can effectively implement the principles of metabolic confusion while maximizing the benefits for your health and well-being.

Start by establishing clear and achievable goals for your Metabolic Confusion Diet journey. Whether you're looking to lose weight, improve energy levels, or optimize your nutritional intake, setting specific, measurable, and realistic goals will help guide your dietary decisions and track your progress over time.

Next, consider how you will incorporate the principles of metabolic confusion into your daily routine. This may involve alternating between higher and lower-calorie days, varying your macronutrient distribution, or experimenting with intermittent fasting protocols. Tailor your approach to suit your lifestyle, preferences, and dietary requirements, keeping in mind that flexibility is key to long-term success.

When crafting your meal plan, focus on incorporating a diverse array of nutrient-dense foods that provide essential vitamins, minerals, and antioxidants. Emphasize whole grains, lean proteins, healthy fats, fruits, and vegetables, while minimizing processed foods, refined sugars, and excessive sodium.

Experiment with new recipes, cooking techniques, and flavor combinations to keep your meals exciting and enjoyable. Don't be afraid to get creative in the kitchen and try new foods – after all, variety is the spice of life!

Finally, monitor your progress regularly and adjust your plan as needed based on feedback from your body and healthcare professionals. Stay mindful of how different dietary choices impact your energy levels, mood, and overall well-being, and be open to making changes as you continue on your Metabolic Confusion Diet journey.

In conclusion, getting started with the Metabolic Confusion Diet requires a thoughtful and personalized approach that takes into account your individual dietary needs, health status, and goals. By assessing your dietary habits, seeking guidance from healthcare professionals, and creating a customized plan tailored to your needs, you can set yourself up for success and embark on a journey towards improved health and vitality.

ESSENTIAL INGREDIENTS ON METABOLIC CONFUSION DIET

Embarking on the Metabolic Confusion Diet is not just about following a set of rules or restrictions; it's about embracing a lifestyle that prioritizes nutrient-dense foods and supports your overall health and well-being. In this chapter, we'll explore the essential ingredients that form the foundation of the Metabolic Confusion Diet, from key nutrients to shopping tips for seniors and strategies for stocking your kitchen for success.

Overview of Key Ingredients

At the heart of the Metabolic Confusion Diet are nutrient-dense ingredients that provide essential vitamins, minerals, antioxidants, and macronutrients to support your body's metabolic processes and overall health. These key ingredients form the building blocks of delicious and nutritious meals that will fuel your body and keep you feeling energized and satisfied.

First and foremost, focus on incorporating plenty of fruits and vegetables into your diet. These colorful gems are packed with vitamins, minerals, fiber, and antioxidants that help support immune function, promote healthy digestion, and reduce the risk of chronic disease. Aim to fill half of your plate with fruits and vegetables at each meal, choosing a variety of colors and textures to maximize nutritional benefits.

Next, prioritize lean proteins such as poultry, fish, eggs, tofu, legumes, and low-fat dairy products. Protein is essential for building and repairing tissues, supporting muscle health, and keeping you feeling full and satisfied between meals. Incorporate protein-rich foods into each meal and snack to help balance blood sugar levels and support healthy metabolism.

Don't forget about healthy fats, which play a crucial role in brain function, hormone production, and nutrient absorption. Include sources of monounsaturated and polyunsaturated fats such as avocados, nuts, seeds, olive oil, and fatty fish in your diet to support heart health and overall well-being. Be mindful of portion sizes, as fats are calorie-dense and can contribute to weight gain if consumed in excess.

Finally, choose whole grains and complex carbohydrates over refined grains and sugars to provide sustained energy and support healthy blood sugar levels. Opt for whole grain bread, brown rice, quinoa, oats, and sweet potatoes, which are rich in fiber, vitamins, and minerals. These wholesome carbohydrates will help keep you feeling full and satisfied while providing essential nutrients to fuel your body.

Shopping Tips for Seniors

Navigating the grocery store can be overwhelming, especially for seniors who may have limited mobility or dietary restrictions. However, with a few simple tips and tricks, you can navigate the aisles with confidence and make informed choices that support your health and well-being.

Start by planning your meals and snacks ahead of time and creating a shopping list based on your meal plan. This will help you stay organized and focused while shopping and prevent impulse purchases of unhealthy foods.

When shopping for fruits and vegetables, choose a variety of fresh, frozen, and canned options to ensure you always have plenty of options on hand. Look for seasonal produce, which is often more affordable and flavorful, and consider purchasing pre-cut or pre-washed fruits and vegetables to save time and effort.

When selecting proteins, opt for lean options such as skinless poultry, fish, eggs, tofu, and legumes. Choose cuts of meat that are low in saturated fat and sodium and look for products labeled "lean" or "extra lean." Consider purchasing frozen or canned proteins, which are convenient and can be stored for longer periods.

When it comes to dairy products, choose low-fat or fat-free options such as skim milk, Greek yogurt, and reduced-fat cheese. Look for products fortified with vitamin D and calcium to support bone health, and consider lactose-free options if you have difficulty digesting dairy.

Stocking Your Kitchen for Success

Creating a kitchen environment that supports your health and well-being is essential for success on the Metabolic Confusion Diet. By stocking your pantry, refrigerator, and freezer with nutritious ingredients, you'll always have healthy options on hand to prepare delicious meals and snacks.

Start by organizing your pantry and refrigerator to make it easy to find healthy ingredients and avoid temptation. Keep fresh fruits and vegetables visible and easily accessible, and store unhealthy snacks and treats out of sight or in hard-to-reach places.

Invest in quality cooking tools and equipment that make meal preparation easier and more enjoyable. Consider purchasing a set of sharp knives, non-stick cookware, and a blender or food processor for preparing smoothies, soups, and sauces.

Stock up on staple ingredients that form the foundation of healthy meals, such as whole grains, legumes, canned tomatoes, broth, herbs and spices, and healthy cooking oils. Keep a variety of nuts, seeds, and dried fruits on hand for quick and nutritious snacks, and consider purchasing shelf-stable protein sources such as canned tuna, beans, and tofu.

Finally, make it a habit to regularly review and replenish your kitchen staples to ensure you always have what you need to prepare healthy and delicious meals. Keep an ongoing shopping list on your refrigerator or smartphone to jot down items as you run out, and schedule regular trips to the grocery store to restock your pantry and refrigerator.

In conclusion, the Metabolic Confusion Diet is built upon a foundation of nutrient-dense ingredients that support your health and well-being. By prioritizing fruits, vegetables, lean proteins, healthy fats, and whole grains, and following these shopping and stocking tips, you'll be well-equipped to embark on a journey towards improved health and vitality.

BREAKFAST RECIPES

Energizing Quinoa Breakfast Bowl

- **Prep Time:** 10 mins
- **Total Time:** 25 mins
- **Servings:** 2 bowls

Ingredients:

- 1/2 cup quinoa, rinsed
- 1 cup water or vegetable broth
- 1 cup spinach leaves
- 1/2 cup cherry tomatoes, halved
- 1/4 cup red onion, diced
- 2 eggs
- Salt and pepper to taste
- Optional: avocado slices, feta cheese crumbles, chopped parsley

Directions:

1. In a medium saucepan, bring the water or vegetable broth to a boil. Add the quinoa, reduce heat to low, cover, and simmer for about 15 minutes or until the quinoa is cooked and the liquid is absorbed.

2. In a separate pan, sauté the spinach, cherry tomatoes, and red onion until the spinach is wilted and the tomatoes are slightly softened.

3. In another pan, fry the eggs to your desired doneness.

4. Divide the cooked quinoa between two bowls. Top each with the sautéed vegetables and a fried egg. Season with salt and pepper to taste.

5. Garnish with avocado slices, feta cheese crumbles, and chopped parsley if desired. Serve hot.

Nutrition Facts (per serving):

- Calories: 319
- Protein: 16g
- Carbohydrates: 38g
- Fat: 12g
- Fiber: 6g

Morning Glory Chia Pudding

- **Prep Time:** 5 mins
- **Total Time:** 4 hours (including chilling time)
- **Servings:** 2 servings

Ingredients:

- 1/4 cup chia seeds
- 1 cup unsweetened almond milk
- 1 tablespoon maple syrup or honey
- 1/2 teaspoon vanilla extract
- 1/2 teaspoon ground cinnamon
- 1/4 cup shredded carrots
- 1/4 cup diced apple
- 2 tablespoons chopped walnuts
- 2 tablespoons unsweetened shredded coconut

Directions:

1. In a mixing bowl, combine the chia seeds, almond milk, maple syrup or honey, vanilla extract, and ground cinnamon. Stir well to combine.

2. Let the mixture sit for 5 minutes, then stir again to prevent clumping. Cover the bowl and refrigerate for at least 4 hours or overnight, allowing the chia seeds to gel and thicken.

3. Once the chia pudding has set, divide it between two serving bowls.

4. Top each bowl with shredded carrots, diced apple, chopped walnuts, and shredded coconut.

5. Serve chilled and enjoy!

Nutrition Facts (per serving):

- Calories: 236
- Protein: 6g
- Carbohydrates: 25g
- Fat: 13g
- Fiber: 10g

Savory Spinach and Mushroom Omelette

- **Prep Time:** 10 mins
- **Total Time:** 15 mins
- **Servings:** 1 omelette

Ingredients:

- 2 large eggs
- 1 tablespoon water
- 1 cup fresh spinach leaves
- 1/2 cup sliced mushrooms

- 1/4 cup diced onion

- 1/4 cup diced bell pepper

- Salt and pepper to taste

- 1 tablespoon olive oil

- Optional: shredded cheese, chopped fresh herbs

Directions:

1. In a small bowl, beat the eggs with the water until well combined. Season with salt and pepper to taste.

2. Heat the olive oil in a non-stick skillet over medium heat. Add the diced onion and bell pepper and sauté until softened, about 2-3 minutes.

3. Add the sliced mushrooms to the skillet and cook until they release their moisture and start to brown, about 3-4 minutes.

4. Add the fresh spinach leaves to the skillet and cook until wilted, about 1-2 minutes.

5. Pour the beaten eggs over the cooked vegetables in the skillet. Use a spatula to gently lift the edges of the omelette and tilt the skillet to allow the uncooked egg mixture to flow underneath.

6. Once the eggs are mostly set but still slightly runny on top, sprinkle the shredded cheese (if using) over one half of the omelette.

7. Use the spatula to fold the other half of the omelette over the cheese, creating a half-moon shape. Press down gently with the spatula to seal.

8. Cook for another 1-2 minutes, or until the cheese is melted and the omelette is cooked through.

9. Slide the omelette onto a plate, garnish with chopped fresh herbs if desired, and serve hot.

Nutrition Facts (per serving):

- Calories: 263
- Protein: 16g
- Carbohydrates: 8g
- Fat: 19g
- Fiber: 3g

High-Protein Greek Yogurt Parfait

- **Prep Time:** 5 mins
- **Total Time:** 5 mins
- **Servings:** 1 parfait

Ingredients:

- 1/2 cup plain Greek yogurt
- 1/4 cup fresh berries (such as strawberries, blueberries, or raspberries)
- 1 tablespoon honey or maple syrup
- 1 tablespoon almond butter or peanut butter
- 2 tablespoons granola
- Optional: sliced banana, chopped nuts, shredded coconut

Directions:

1. In a serving glass or bowl, layer the plain Greek yogurt, fresh berries, honey or maple syrup, almond butter or peanut butter, and granola.
2. Repeat the layers until all ingredients are used, ending with a sprinkle of granola on top.

3. Garnish with sliced banana, chopped nuts, and shredded coconut if desired.

4. Serve immediately and enjoy!

Nutrition Facts (per serving):

- Calories: 342

- Protein: 17g

- Carbohydrates: 44g

- Fat: 13g

- Fiber: 5g

Avocado and Spinach Breakfast Wrap

- **Prep Time:** 5 mins

- **Total Time:** 10 mins

- **Servings:** 1 wrap

Ingredients:

- 1 whole grain or gluten-free wrap

- 1/2 avocado, mashed

- 1/2 cup fresh spinach leaves

- 1/4 cup diced tomatoes

- 2 eggs, scrambled

- Salt and pepper to taste

- Optional: salsa, hot sauce, shredded cheese

Directions:

1. Heat the whole grain or gluten-free wrap in a dry skillet over medium heat for about 1 minute on each side, until warm and slightly toasted.

2. Spread the mashed avocado evenly over the warmed wrap.

3. Layer the fresh spinach leaves and diced tomatoes on top of the mashed avocado.

4. In a separate pan, scramble the eggs until cooked through. Season with salt and pepper to taste.

5. Spoon the scrambled eggs onto the wrap over the spinach and tomatoes.

6. Optional: Add salsa, hot sauce, or shredded cheese for extra flavor.

7. Roll up the wrap tightly, slice in half if desired, and serve immediately.

Nutrition Facts (per serving):

- Calories: 345
- Protein: 17g
- Carbohydrates: 24g
- Fat: 20g
- Fiber: 9g

Quinoa Breakfast Bowl

- **Prep Time:** 5 mins
- **Total Time:** 20 mins
- **Servings:** 2 bowls

Ingredients:

- 1/2 cup quinoa, rinsed
- 1 cup water or vegetable broth
- 1/2 cup diced bell pepper
- 1/4 cup diced red onion
- 1/2 cup black beans, drained and rinsed

- 1/2 avocado, sliced
- 2 eggs, poached or fried
- Salt and pepper to taste
- Optional: salsa, cilantro, lime wedges

Directions:

1. In a medium saucepan, bring the water or vegetable broth to a boil. Add the quinoa, reduce heat to low, cover, and simmer for about 15 minutes or until the quinoa is cooked and the liquid is absorbed.
2. In a separate pan, sauté the diced bell pepper and red onion until softened, about 3-4 minutes.
3. Add the black beans to the pan with the sautéed vegetables and cook for an additional 2-3 minutes, until heated through.
4. Divide the cooked quinoa between two bowls. Top each with the sautéed vegetables, sliced avocado, and a poached or fried egg.
5. Season with salt and pepper to taste. Serve with optional salsa, cilantro, and lime wedges on the side.

Nutrition Facts (per serving):

- Calories: 372
- Protein: 18g
- Carbohydrates: 40g
- Fat: 17g
- Fiber: 10g

Greek Yogurt Berry Parfait

- **Prep Time:** 5 mins

- **Total Time:** 5 mins
- **Servings:** 1 parfait

Ingredients:

- 1/2 cup plain Greek yogurt
- 1/4 cup granola
- 1/4 cup mixed berries (such as strawberries, blueberries, raspberries)
- 1 tablespoon honey or maple syrup
- Optional: sliced banana, chopped nuts, shredded coconut

Directions:

1. In a serving glass or bowl, layer the plain Greek yogurt, granola, and mixed berries.
2. Drizzle honey or maple syrup over the berries.
3. Repeat the layers until all ingredients are used, ending with a sprinkle of granola on top.
4. Garnish with sliced banana, chopped nuts, and shredded coconut if desired.
5. Serve immediately and enjoy!

Nutrition Facts (per serving):

- Calories: 290
- Protein: 16g
- Carbohydrates: 46g
- Fat: 6g
- Fiber: 6g

Sweet Potato and Spinach Breakfast Hash

- **Prep Time:** 10 mins

- **Total Time:** 25 mins
- **Servings:** 2 servings

Ingredients:

- 1 large sweet potato, diced
- 1 tablespoon olive oil
- 1/2 cup diced onion
- 1 clove garlic, minced
- 2 cups fresh spinach leaves
- 1/4 teaspoon paprika
- Salt and pepper to taste
- 2 eggs
- Optional: chopped fresh parsley, hot sauce

Directions:

1. Heat the olive oil in a large skillet over medium heat. Add the diced sweet potato and cook for about 10-12 minutes, stirring occasionally, until tender and golden brown.
2. Add the diced onion and minced garlic to the skillet with the sweet potato. Cook for an additional 2-3 minutes until the onion is softened and translucent.
3. Add the fresh spinach leaves to the skillet and cook until wilted, about 1-2 minutes.
4. Season the hash with paprika, salt, and pepper to taste. Stir to combine.
5. Make two wells in the hash and crack an egg into each well.
6. Cover the skillet and cook for about 3-4 minutes, or until the eggs are cooked to your desired doneness.

7. Garnish with chopped fresh parsley and hot sauce if desired. Serve hot.

Nutrition Facts (per serving):

- Calories: 275
- Protein: 11g
- Carbohydrates: 30g
- Fat: 13g
- Fiber: 5g

Spinach & Egg Scramble with Raspberries

- **Prep Time:** 11 mins,
- **Total Time:** 11 mins,
- **Servings:** 1, Yield: 1 serving

Ingredients

- 1 tsp canola oil
- 1 1/2 cups baby spinach
- 2 large eggs, lightly beaten
- Pinch kosher salt
- Pinch ground pepper
- 1 slice whole-grain bread, toasted
- 1/2 cup fresh raspberries

Directions

1. In a nonstick skillet over medium-high, heat oil. Sauté spinach until wilted, 1-2 mins. Remove and set aside.

2. In the same skillet over medium, cook eggs, stirring, until set, 1-2 mins. Combine with spinach, season with salt and pepper. Serve with toast and raspberries.

Nutrition Facts (per serving)

- Calories: 297.1
- Fat: 16.1g
- Carbs: 21.1g
- Protein: 18.1g

Protein-Packed Breakfast Smoothie Bowl

Prep Time: 5 mins

Total Time: 5 mins

Servings: 1 bowl

Ingredients:

- 1 ripe banana, frozen
- 1/2 cup frozen berries (such as strawberries, blueberries, raspberries)
- 1/2 cup plain Greek yogurt
- 1/4 cup unsweetened almond milk
- 1 tablespoon almond butter or peanut butter
- 1 tablespoon chia seeds
- Optional toppings: sliced almonds, shredded coconut, fresh berries, granola

Directions:

1. In a blender, combine the frozen banana, frozen berries, plain Greek yogurt, unsweetened almond milk, almond butter or peanut butter, and chia seeds.
2. Blend on high until smooth and creamy, adding more almond milk if needed to reach your desired consistency.
3. Pour the smoothie into a bowl.

4. Top with optional toppings such as sliced almonds, shredded coconut, fresh berries, and granola.

5. Serve immediately and enjoy!

Nutrition Facts (per serving):

- Calories: 406
- Protein: 24g
- Carbohydrates: 49g
- Fat: 16g
- Fiber: 11g

Vegetable and Egg Breakfast Casserole

Prep Time: 15 mins

Total Time: 45 mins

Servings: 4 servings

Ingredients:

- 6 eggs
- 1/4 cup milk or unsweetened almond milk
- 1 cup chopped vegetables (such as bell peppers, onions, spinach)
- 1/2 cup shredded cheese
- Salt and pepper to taste
- Optional: cooked quinoa or brown rice

Directions:

1. Preheat your oven to 350°F (175°C). Grease a baking dish with cooking spray.

2. In a mixing bowl, whisk together the eggs and milk until well combined. Season with salt and pepper.

3. Stir in the chopped vegetables and shredded cheese.

4. Pour the egg mixture into the prepared baking dish.

5. Bake for 30-35 minutes, or until the eggs are set and the top is golden brown.

6. Remove from the oven and let cool for a few minutes before slicing.

7. Serve the breakfast casserole warm, with optional cooked quinoa or brown rice on the side if desired.

Nutrition Facts (per serving):

- Calories: 218

- Protein: 16g

- Carbohydrates: 6g

- Fat: 14g

- Fiber: 1g

Pineapple Green Smoothie

- **Prep Time:** 6 mins,

- **Total Time:** 6 mins,

- **Servings:** 1,

- **Yield:** 1 serving

Ingredients

- 1/2 cup almond milk, unsweetened

- 1/3 cup Greek yogurt, nonfat plain

- 1 cup baby spinach

- 1 cup frozen banana slices

- 1/2 cup frozen pineapple chunks

- 1 tbsp chia seeds

- 1-2 tsp maple syrup or honey (optional)

Directions

1. Blend almond milk and yogurt with spinach, banana, pineapple, chia seeds, and sweetener (if used) until smooth.

Nutrition Facts (per serving)

- Calories: 297.6
- Fat: 6.1g
- Carbs: 54.1g
- Protein: 13.1g

Nutty Banana Breakfast Bowl

Prep Time: 5 mins

Total Time: 10 mins

Servings: 1 bowl

Ingredients:

- 1 ripe banana
- 1/4 cup rolled oats
- 1 tablespoon almond butter or peanut butter
- 1 tablespoon chia seeds
- 1/2 cup unsweetened almond milk
- 1/4 teaspoon cinnamon
- Optional toppings: sliced almonds, shredded coconut, fresh berries, honey or maple syrup

Directions:

1. In a microwave-safe bowl, mash the ripe banana with a fork until smooth.

2. Add the rolled oats, almond butter or peanut butter, chia seeds, unsweetened almond milk, and cinnamon to the bowl.

3. Stir until all ingredients are well combined.

4. Microwave on high for 1-2 minutes, or until the mixture is heated through and the oats are cooked.

5. Stir the mixture again, then let it sit for a few minutes to thicken.

6. Top with optional toppings such as sliced almonds, shredded coconut, fresh berries, and a drizzle of honey or maple syrup.

7. Serve warm and enjoy!

Nutrition Facts (per serving):

- Calories: 367
- Protein: 9g
- Carbohydrates: 56g
- Fat: 14g
- Fiber: 11g

Egg and Veggie Breakfast Muffins

Prep Time: 10 mins

Total Time: 25 mins

Servings: 6 muffins

Ingredients:

- 6 eggs
- 1/4 cup milk or unsweetened almond milk
- 1 cup chopped vegetables (such as bell peppers, spinach, mushrooms)
- 1/4 cup shredded cheese

- Salt and pepper to taste
- Optional: chopped cooked bacon or sausage

Directions:

1. Preheat your oven to 350°F (175°C). Grease a muffin tin with cooking spray or line with paper liners.
2. In a mixing bowl, whisk together the eggs and milk until well combined. Season with salt and pepper.
3. Stir in the chopped vegetables, shredded cheese, and optional chopped cooked bacon or sausage.
4. Divide the egg mixture evenly among the muffin cups, filling each about 3/4 full.
5. Bake for 15-20 minutes, or until the eggs are set and the tops are golden brown.
6. Remove from the oven and let cool for a few minutes before removing from the muffin tin.
7. Serve the breakfast muffins warm or at room temperature.

Nutrition Facts (per serving - 1 muffin):

- Calories: 120
- Protein: 9g
- Carbohydrates: 3g
- Fat: 8g
- Fiber: 1g

SNACKS RECIPES

Savory Chickpea Snack

- **Prep Time:** 5 mins

  Total Time: 20 mins

  Servings: 4 servings

Ingredients:

- 1 can (15 ounces) chickpeas, drained and rinsed
- 1 tablespoon olive oil
- 1 teaspoon ground cumin
- 1/2 teaspoon paprika
- 1/2 teaspoon garlic powder
- Salt and pepper to taste

Directions:

1. Preheat your oven to 400°F (200°C). Line a baking sheet with parchment paper.
2. In a mixing bowl, toss the chickpeas with olive oil, ground cumin, paprika, garlic powder, salt, and pepper until evenly coated.
3. Spread the seasoned chickpeas in a single layer on the prepared baking sheet.
4. Bake for 15-20 minutes, stirring halfway through, until the chickpeas are golden and crispy.
5. Remove from the oven and let cool slightly before serving.
6. Enjoy as a crunchy and satisfying snack!

Nutrition Facts (per serving):

- Calories: 116
- Protein: 5g
- Carbohydrates: 16g
- Fat: 4g
- Fiber: 5g

Greek Yogurt and Fruit Parfait

- **Prep Time:** 5 mins

  Total Time: 5 mins

  Servings: 1 serving

Ingredients:

- 1/2 cup plain Greek yogurt
- 1/4 cup granola
- 1/4 cup mixed berries (such as strawberries, blueberries, raspberries)
- Optional: honey or maple syrup for sweetness

Directions:

1. In a serving glass or bowl, layer the plain Greek yogurt, granola, and mixed berries.
2. Drizzle with honey or maple syrup if desired for extra sweetness.
3. Repeat the layers until all ingredients are used.
4. Serve immediately and enjoy this refreshing snack!

Nutrition Facts (per serving):

- Calories: 230
- Protein: 14g
- Carbohydrates: 32g

- Fat: 6g

- Fiber: 4g

Cucumber and Hummus Bites

- **Prep Time:** 10 mins

  Total Time: 10 mins

  Servings: 2 servings

Ingredients:

- 1 large cucumber

- 1/2 cup hummus

- Optional toppings: cherry tomatoes, olives, fresh herbs

Directions:

1. Wash the cucumber and cut it into thick slices.

2. Use a small spoon or melon baller to scoop out some of the seeds from each cucumber slice, creating a small well in the center.

3. Spoon a dollop of hummus into each cucumber well.

4. Garnish with optional toppings such as halved cherry tomatoes, sliced olives, or chopped fresh herbs.

5. Serve immediately and enjoy this refreshing and crunchy snack!

Nutrition Facts (per serving):

- Calories: 105

- Protein: 5g

- Carbohydrates: 13g

- Fat: 5g

- Fiber: 5g

Turkey and Cheese Roll-Ups

- **Prep Time:** 10 mins

  Total Time: 10 mins

  Servings: 2 servings

Ingredients:

- 4 slices deli turkey or chicken breast
- 2 slices cheese (such as cheddar or Swiss)
- 1/2 avocado, thinly sliced
- Optional: mustard, mayonnaise, lettuce leaves

Directions:

1. Lay out the slices of deli turkey or chicken breast on a clean surface.
2. Place a slice of cheese on top of each slice of turkey.
3. Add a few slices of avocado on top of the cheese.
4. Optional: Spread mustard or mayonnaise on top of the avocado, and top with a lettuce leaf.
5. Roll up each slice tightly to create a roll-up.
6. Secure with toothpicks if necessary.
7. Serve immediately and enjoy this protein-packed snack!

Nutrition Facts (per serving):

- Calories: 218
- Protein: 17g
- Carbohydrates: 4g
- Fat: 16g
- Fiber: 3g

Smashed Avocado Rice Cakes

- **Prep Time:** 5 mins

  Total Time: 5 mins

  Servings: 2 servings

Ingredients:

- 2 rice cakes
- 1 ripe avocado
- 1/2 lemon, juiced
- Salt and pepper to taste
- Optional toppings: cherry tomatoes, sliced cucumber, red pepper flakes

Directions:

1. Cut the avocado in half, remove the pit, and scoop the flesh into a small bowl.
2. Add lemon juice, salt, and pepper to the bowl.
3. Use a fork to mash the avocado until smooth and well combined with the lemon juice and seasonings.
4. Spread the smashed avocado evenly onto each rice cake.
5. Top with optional toppings such as sliced cherry tomatoes, cucumber, or a sprinkle of red pepper flakes.
6. Serve immediately and enjoy this quick and satisfying snack!

Nutrition Facts (per serving):

- Calories: 138
- Protein: 2g
- Carbohydrates: 9g
- Fat: 11g
- Fiber: 4g

Apple Slices with Almond Butter

- **Prep Time:** 5 mins

  Total Time: 5 mins

  Servings: 2 servings

Ingredients:

- 1 apple, sliced
- 2 tablespoons almond butter
- Optional toppings: cinnamon, shredded coconut, sliced almonds

Directions:

1. Wash and slice the apple into thin wedges.
2. Spread almond butter onto each apple slice.
3. Sprinkle with optional toppings such as cinnamon, shredded coconut, or sliced almonds.
4. Serve immediately and enjoy this crunchy and nutritious snack!

Nutrition Facts (per serving):

- Calories: 180
- Protein: 4g
- Carbohydrates: 19g
- Fat: 11g
- Fiber: 5g

Crispy Kale Chips

- **Prep Time:** 10 mins

  Total Time: 20 mins

  Servings: 2 servings

Ingredients:

- 1 bunch kale
- 1 tablespoon olive oil
- Salt and pepper to taste
- Optional: nutritional yeast, garlic powder, chili powder

Directions:

1. Preheat your oven to 350°F (175°C). Line a baking sheet with parchment paper.
2. Wash the kale leaves and thoroughly dry them with a kitchen towel or salad spinner.
3. Remove the tough stems from the kale leaves and tear them into bite-sized pieces.
4. In a large bowl, toss the kale pieces with olive oil, salt, and pepper until evenly coated.
5. Spread the kale pieces in a single layer on the prepared baking sheet.
6. Bake for 10-15 minutes, or until the kale is crispy and slightly browned, stirring halfway through.
7. Remove from the oven and let cool for a few minutes before serving.
8. Sprinkle with optional toppings such as nutritional yeast, garlic powder, or chili powder.
9. Enjoy these crispy and flavorful kale chips as a nutritious snack!

Nutrition Facts (per serving):

- Calories: 64
- Protein: 2g

- Carbohydrates: 4g
- Fat: 4g
- Fiber: 1g

Berry and Nut Trail Mix

- **Prep Time:** 5 mins

  Total Time: 5 mins

  Servings: 4 servings

Ingredients:

- 1/2 cup mixed nuts (such as almonds, walnuts, cashews)
- 1/4 cup dried cranberries
- 1/4 cup freeze-dried strawberries
- 1/4 cup dark chocolate chips or chunks

Directions:

1. In a mixing bowl, combine the mixed nuts, dried cranberries, freeze-dried strawberries, and dark chocolate chips.
2. Toss until all ingredients are evenly distributed.
3. Divide the trail mix into individual serving portions.
4. Pack in small resalable bags or containers for easy grab-and-go snacks.
5. Enjoy this sweet and savory trail mix whenever you need a quick energy boost!

Nutrition Facts (per serving):

- Calories: 154
- Protein: 4g
- Carbohydrates: 13g
- Fat: 10g

- Fiber: 2g

Hummus and Veggie Dip

- **Prep Time:** 10 mins

  Total Time: 10 mins

  Servings: 4 servings

Ingredients:

- 1 cup hummus
- Assorted veggies for dipping (carrots, cucumber, bell peppers, cherry tomatoes)

Directions:

1. Transfer the hummus to a serving bowl.
2. Wash and prepare the assorted veggies by slicing them into sticks or bite-sized pieces.
3. Arrange the veggie sticks around the bowl of hummus for dipping.
4. Serve immediately and enjoy this nutritious and satisfying snack!

Nutrition Facts (per serving):

- Calories: 143
- Protein: 6g
- Carbohydrates: 16g
- Fat: 6g
- Fiber: 5g

Turkey and Cheese Roll-Ups

- **Prep Time:** 5 mins

  Total Time: 5 mins

  Servings: 2 servings

Ingredients:

- 4 slices deli turkey or chicken breast
- 2 slices cheese (such as cheddar or Swiss)
- Optional: mustard, mayonnaise, lettuce leaves

Directions:

1. Lay out the slices of deli turkey or chicken breast on a clean surface.
2. Place a slice of cheese on top of each slice of turkey.
3. Optional: Spread mustard or mayonnaise on top of the cheese, and top with a lettuce leaf.
4. Roll up each slice tightly to create a roll-up.
5. Serve immediately and enjoy this protein-packed snack!

Nutrition Facts (per serving):

- Calories: 218
- Protein: 17g
- Carbohydrates: 4g
- Fat: 16g
- Fiber: 3g

Nutty Yogurt Dip with Fruit Slices

- **Prep Time:** 5 mins

  Total Time: 5 mins

  Servings: 2 servings

Ingredients:

- 1/2 cup Greek yogurt
- 2 tablespoons almond butter or peanut butter
- 1 tablespoon honey or maple syrup
- 1/2 teaspoon vanilla extract
- Assorted fruit slices for dipping (such as apple, pear, banana, strawberries)

Directions:

1. In a small bowl, combine the Greek yogurt, almond butter or peanut butter, honey or maple syrup, and vanilla extract. Mix until smooth.
2. Wash and prepare the assorted fruit by slicing them into bite-sized pieces.
3. Transfer the nutty yogurt dip to a serving bowl and arrange the fruit slices around it for dipping.
4. Serve immediately and enjoy this delicious and protein-rich snack!

Nutrition Facts (per serving):

- Calories: 196
- Protein: 9g
- Carbohydrates: 21g
- Fat: 9g
- Fiber: 3g

Quinoa and Veggie Stuffed Bell Peppers

- **Prep Time:** 10 mins

  Total Time: 30 mins

  Servings: 2 servings

Ingredients:

- 1/2 cup cooked quinoa
- 1/2 cup mixed veggies (such as diced bell peppers, onions, zucchini)
- 1/4 cup shredded cheese
- 2 large bell peppers, halved and deseeded
- Salt and pepper to taste
- Optional: chopped fresh herbs (such as parsley or basil)

Directions:

1. Preheat your oven to 375°F (190°C). Line a baking dish with parchment paper.
2. In a mixing bowl, combine the cooked quinoa, mixed veggies, shredded cheese, salt, and pepper. Mix until well combined.
3. Stuff each bell pepper half with the quinoa and veggie mixture.
4. Place the stuffed bell peppers in the prepared baking dish.
5. Bake for 20-25 minutes, or until the peppers are tender and the filling is heated through.
6. Remove from the oven and let cool for a few minutes before serving.
7. Garnish with optional chopped fresh herbs before serving.
8. Enjoy these flavorful and nutritious stuffed bell peppers as a satisfying snack!

Nutrition Facts (per serving):

- Calories: 204
- Protein: 10g
- Carbohydrates: 24g

- Fat: 8g

- Fiber: 6g

Nutty Banana Slices

- **Prep Time:** 5 mins

  Total Time: 5 mins

  Servings: 2 servings

Ingredients:

- 1 large banana, peeled and sliced

- 2 tablespoons almond butter or peanut butter

- Optional toppings: chia seeds, shredded coconut, cinnamon

Directions:

1. Arrange the banana slices on a serving plate or cutting board.

2. Spread a dollop of almond butter or peanut butter on each banana slice.

3. Sprinkle with optional toppings such as chia seeds, shredded coconut, or cinnamon.

4. Serve immediately and enjoy this simple and satisfying snack!

Nutrition Facts (per serving):

- Calories: 191

- Protein: 4g

- Carbohydrates: 20g

- Fat: 11g

- Fiber: 3g

Veggie Sticks with Hummus

- **Prep Time:** 10 mins

  Total Time: 10 mins

  Servings: 2 servings

Ingredients:

- Assorted veggies for dipping (carrots, cucumber, bell peppers)
- 1/2 cup hummus

Directions:

1. Wash and prepare the assorted veggies by slicing them into sticks or bite-sized pieces.
2. Transfer the hummus to a serving bowl.
3. Arrange the veggie sticks around the bowl of hummus for dipping.
4. Serve immediately and enjoy this crunchy and nutritious snack!

Nutrition Facts (per serving):

- Calories: 142
- Protein: 6g
- Carbohydrates: 15g
- Fat: 7g
- Fiber: 5g

Cucumber and Cottage Cheese Boats

- **Prep Time:** 10 mins

  Total Time: 10 mins

  Servings: 2 servings

Ingredients:

- 1 large cucumber
- 1/2 cup low-fat cottage cheese

- 1 tablespoon chopped fresh dill or parsley
- Salt and pepper to taste

Directions:

1. Wash the cucumber and cut it in half lengthwise.
2. Use a spoon to scoop out the seeds and create a hollow center in each cucumber half.
3. In a small bowl, mix the cottage cheese with chopped fresh dill or parsley, salt, and pepper.
4. Spoon the cottage cheese mixture into the hollowed-out center of each cucumber half.
5. Serve immediately and enjoy this refreshing and protein-packed snack!

Nutrition Facts (per serving):

- Calories: 85
- Protein: 9g
- Carbohydrates: 7g
- Fat: 3g
- Fiber: 1g

Egg Salad Stuffed Celery

- **Prep Time:** 10 mins

  Total Time: 10 mins

  Servings: 2 servings

Ingredients:

- 2 large celery stalks
- 2 hard-boiled eggs, chopped
- 2 tablespoons Greek yogurt or mayonnaise

- 1 tablespoon chopped chives or green onions
- Salt and pepper to taste

Directions:

1. Wash the celery stalks and cut them into manageable lengths.
2. In a mixing bowl, combine the chopped hard-boiled eggs, Greek yogurt or mayonnaise, chopped chives or green onions, salt, and pepper.
3. Mix until well combined.
4. Spoon the egg salad mixture into the hollowed-out center of each celery stalk.
5. Serve immediately and enjoy this crunchy and satisfying snack!

Nutrition Facts (per serving):

- Calories: 112
- Protein: 10g
- Carbohydrates: 3g
- Fat: 7g
- Fiber: 1g

BEVERAGES RECIPES

Green Tea Lemonade

- **Prep Time:** 5 mins

  Total Time: 10 mins

  Servings: 2 servings

Ingredients:

- 2 cups water
- 2 green tea bags
- 1 lemon, juiced
- 1 tablespoon honey or maple syrup
- Ice cubes
- Optional: fresh mint leaves for garnish

Directions:

1. Bring the water to a boil in a saucepan.
2. Remove from heat and add the green tea bags. Let steep for 5 minutes.
3. Remove the tea bags and allow the tea to cool to room temperature.
4. Once cooled, stir in the lemon juice and honey or maple syrup.
5. Fill two glasses with ice cubes.
6. Pour the green tea lemonade over the ice cubes.
7. Garnish with fresh mint leaves if desired.
8. Serve immediately and enjoy this refreshing and antioxidant-rich beverage!

Nutrition Facts (per serving):

- Calories: 22
- Protein: 0g
- Carbohydrates: 6g
- Fat: 0g
- Fiber: 0g

Berry Protein Smoothie

- **Prep Time:** 5 mins

  Total Time: 5 mins

  Servings: 2 servings

Ingredients:

- 1 cup frozen mixed berries (such as strawberries, blueberries, raspberries)
- 1/2 cup plain Greek yogurt
- 1/2 cup unsweetened almond milk
- 1 scoop protein powder (vanilla or berry-flavored)
- 1 tablespoon chia seeds
- Ice cubes

Directions:

1. In a blender, combine the frozen mixed berries, Greek yogurt, almond milk, protein powder, and chia seeds.
2. Blend until smooth and creamy.
3. If the smoothie is too thick, add more almond milk until desired consistency is reached.
4. Add ice cubes to the blender and pulse until crushed and incorporated into the smoothie.
5. Pour into glasses and serve immediately.

6. Enjoy this protein-packed smoothie as a nutritious and energizing beverage!

Nutrition Facts (per serving):

- Calories: 185
- Protein: 19g
- Carbohydrates: 16g
- Fat: 6g
- Fiber: 6g

Turmeric Ginger Tea

- **Prep Time:** 5 mins

  Total Time: 10 mins

  Servings: 2 servings

Ingredients:

- 2 cups water
- 1 teaspoon ground turmeric
- 1 teaspoon grated fresh ginger
- 1 tablespoon honey or maple syrup (optional)
- Juice of 1/2 lemon
- Pinch of black pepper

Directions:

1. In a small saucepan, bring the water to a boil.
2. Add the ground turmeric and grated ginger to the boiling water.
3. Reduce the heat to low and let the mixture simmer for 5 minutes.
4. Remove the saucepan from heat and strain the tea into mugs.

5. Stir in honey or maple syrup if desired, and add a squeeze of lemon juice.

6. Sprinkle with a pinch of black pepper.

7. Serve immediately and enjoy this soothing and immune-boosting beverage!

Nutrition Facts (per serving):

- Calories: 16
- Protein: 0g
- Carbohydrates: 4g
- Fat: 0g
- Fiber: 0g

Vanilla Almond Milkshake

- **Prep Time:** 5 mins

  Total Time: 5 mins

  Servings: 2 servings

Ingredients:

- 2 cups unsweetened almond milk
- 1/2 teaspoon vanilla extract
- 1 tablespoon almond butter
- 1 tablespoon honey or maple syrup (optional)
- Ice cubes

Directions:

1. In a blender, combine the unsweetened almond milk, vanilla extract, almond butter, and honey or maple syrup if using.

2. Blend until smooth and creamy.

3. Add ice cubes to the blender and pulse until crushed and incorporated into the milkshake.

4. Pour into glasses and serve immediately.

5. Enjoy this delicious and protein-rich beverage as a satisfying snack or dessert alternative!

Nutrition Facts (per serving):

- Calories: 92
- Protein: 3g
- Carbohydrates: 4g
- Fat: 7g
- Fiber: 1g

Matcha Protein Smoothie

- **Prep Time:** 5 mins

    Total Time: 5 mins

    Servings: 2 servings

Ingredients:

- 1 cup unsweetened almond milk
- 1 tablespoon matcha powder
- 1 scoop vanilla protein powder
- 1/2 banana, frozen
- 1 tablespoon almond butter
- Ice cubes

Directions:

1. In a blender, combine unsweetened almond milk, matcha powder, vanilla protein powder, frozen banana, and almond butter.

2. Blend until smooth.

3. Add ice cubes and blend again until desired consistency is reached.

4. Pour into glasses and serve immediately.

5. Enjoy this energizing and antioxidant-rich smoothie as a satisfying beverage or post-workout snack!

Nutrition Facts (per serving):

- Calories: 190
- Protein: 20g
- Carbohydrates: 13g
- Fat: 7g
- Fiber: 4g

Turmeric Latte

- **Prep Time:** 2 mins
  Total Time: 7 mins
  Servings: 2 servings

Ingredients:

- 2 cups unsweetened almond milk
- 1 teaspoon ground turmeric
- 1/2 teaspoon ground cinnamon
- 1/4 teaspoon ground ginger
- 1 tablespoon honey or maple syrup (optional)
- Pinch of black pepper

Directions:

1. In a small saucepan, heat the unsweetened almond milk over medium heat.

2. Whisk in ground turmeric, ground cinnamon, and ground ginger.

3. Let the mixture simmer for 5 minutes, stirring occasionally.

4. Remove from heat and stir in honey or maple syrup if desired.

5. Pour into mugs and sprinkle with a pinch of black pepper.

6. Serve immediately and enjoy this comforting and anti-inflammatory beverage!

Nutrition Facts (per serving):

- Calories: 50
- Protein: 1g
- Carbohydrates: 8g
- Fat: 2g
- Fiber: 1g

Green Goddess Smoothie

- **Prep Time:** 5 mins
  Total Time: 5 mins
  Servings: 2 servings

Ingredients:

- 1 cup frozen organic blueberries or mixed berries
- 1/2 cup ice made with filtered or spring water
- 1 cup coconut water or almond milk
- 1 1/2 cups mixed greens (kale, spinach, lettuce)
- 1/2 avocado
- 1 tablespoon chia seeds
- 1 teaspoon honey or maple syrup (optional)
- Optional: 1 scoop protein powder

Directions:

1. In a blender, combine the frozen berries, ice, coconut water or almond milk, mixed greens, avocado, chia seeds, and honey or maple syrup.

2. Optionally, add a scoop of protein powder for extra protein.

3. Blend until smooth and creamy.

4. Pour into glasses and serve immediately.

5. Enjoy this nutrient-packed smoothie to kickstart your day!

Nutrition Facts (per serving):

- Calories: 195
- Protein: 5g
- Carbohydrates: 22g
- Fat: 10g
- Fiber: 7g

Turmeric Golden Milk

- **Prep Time:** 5 mins

  Total Time: 10 mins

  Servings: 2 servings

Ingredients:

- 2 cups unsweetened almond milk or coconut milk
- 1 teaspoon ground turmeric
- 1/2 teaspoon ground cinnamon
- 1/4 teaspoon ground ginger
- Pinch of black pepper
- 1 teaspoon honey or maple syrup (optional)

Directions:

1. In a small saucepan, heat the almond milk or coconut milk over medium heat.
2. Stir in the ground turmeric, cinnamon, ginger, and black pepper.
3. Heat the mixture until it just starts to simmer, then reduce the heat to low.
4. Let the golden milk simmer for 5 minutes, stirring occasionally.
5. Remove from heat and stir in honey or maple syrup if desired.
6. Pour into mugs and serve warm.
7. Enjoy this comforting and anti-inflammatory beverage!

Nutrition Facts (per serving):

- Calories: 45
- Protein: 1g
- Carbohydrates: 3g
- Fat: 3g
- Fiber: 1g

Green Energy Boost Smoothie

- **Prep Time:** 5 mins

  Total Time: 5 mins

  Servings: 2 glasses

Ingredients:

- 1 cup frozen organic blueberries or mixed berries
- 1/2 cup ice made with filtered or spring water
- 1 cup coconut water or almond milk
- 1 1/2 cups mixed greens (kale, spinach, lettuce)
- 1/2 avocado
- 1 tablespoon chia seeds

- 1 teaspoon honey or maple syrup (optional)
- Optional: 1 scoop protein powder

Directions:

1. Place frozen berries, ice, coconut water or almond milk, mixed greens, avocado, chia seeds, and honey or maple syrup in a blender.
2. Add a scoop of protein powder for additional protein if desired.
3. Blend until smooth and creamy.
4. Pour into glasses and serve immediately.
5. Enjoy this refreshing and energizing smoothie as a nutrient-packed snack or meal replacement!

Nutrition Facts (per serving):

- Calories: 210
- Protein: 6g
- Carbohydrates: 26g
- Fat: 10g
- Fiber: 10g

Turmeric Ginger Lemonade

- **Prep Time:** 5 mins
  Total Time: 10 mins
  Servings: 2 glasses

Ingredients:

- 2 cups filtered water
- 1-inch piece of fresh ginger, grated
- 1 teaspoon ground turmeric
- Juice of 1 lemon

- 1-2 tablespoons honey or maple syrup (adjust to taste)
- Ice cubes

Directions:

1. In a small saucepan, bring water to a boil.
2. Add grated ginger and ground turmeric to the boiling water. Let simmer for 5 minutes.
3. Remove from heat and let cool slightly.
4. Stir in lemon juice and honey or maple syrup.
5. Allow the mixture to cool completely, then strain to remove ginger pieces.
6. Serve over ice cubes in glasses.
7. Enjoy this refreshing and immune-boosting lemonade!

Nutrition Facts (per serving):

- Calories: 30
- Protein: 0g
- Carbohydrates: 8g
- Fat: 0g
- Fiber: 0g

Detoxifying Green Tea Lemonade

- **Prep Time:** 5 mins

  Total Time: 10 mins

  Servings: 2 glasses

Ingredients:

- 2 cups water
- 2 green tea bags
- Juice of 1 lemon

- 1 tablespoon honey or maple syrup (optional)
- Ice cubes
- Fresh mint leaves for garnish (optional)

Directions:

1. Bring water to a boil in a small saucepan. Remove from heat and add green tea bags. Let steep for 3-5 minutes.
2. Remove the tea bags and allow the tea to cool to room temperature.
3. Stir in the lemon juice and honey or maple syrup, if using.
4. Chill the lemonade in the refrigerator or pour over ice cubes.
5. Garnish with fresh mint leaves if desired.
6. Serve and enjoy this refreshing and detoxifying beverage!

Nutrition Facts (per serving):

- Calories: 10
- Protein: 0g
- Carbohydrates: 3g
- Fat: 0g
- Fiber: 0g

Cucumber Mint Infused Water

- **Prep Time:** 5 mins
  Total Time: 5 mins
  Servings: 2 glasses

Ingredients:

- 2 cups filtered water
- 1/2 cucumber, thinly sliced
- 6-8 fresh mint leaves

- Ice cubes

Directions:

1. In a pitcher, combine filtered water, cucumber slices, and fresh mint leaves.
2. Stir well and refrigerate for at least 30 minutes to allow the flavors to infuse.
3. Pour the infused water into glasses over ice cubes.
4. Serve and enjoy this hydrating and refreshing beverage!

Nutrition Facts (per serving):

- Calories: 0
- Protein: 0g
- Carbohydrates: 0g
- Fat: 0g
- Fiber: 0g

Berry Blast Smoothie Bowl

- **Prep Time:** 10 mins

    Total Time: 10 mins

    Servings: 2 bowls

Ingredients:

- 1 cup frozen mixed berries
- 1 ripe banana
- 1/2 cup unsweetened almond milk
- 1 tablespoon chia seeds
- Toppings: sliced fresh berries, shredded coconut, granola, nuts/seeds

Directions:

1. In a blender, combine frozen mixed berries, banana, almond milk, and chia seeds.

2. Blend until smooth and creamy.

3. Pour the smoothie into bowls.

4. Top with sliced fresh berries, shredded coconut, granola, and nuts/seeds.

5. Serve immediately and enjoy this delicious and nutritious smoothie bowl!

Nutrition Facts (per serving):

- Calories: 180
- Protein: 4g
- Carbohydrates: 35g
- Fat: 4g
- Fiber: 9g

Green Goddess Smoothie

- **Prep Time:** 5 mins

  Total Time: 5 mins

  Servings: 2 glasses

Ingredients:

- 1 cup spinach leaves
- 1 cup kale leaves, stems removed
- 1/2 cup frozen mango chunks
- 1/2 avocado
- 1 tablespoon chia seeds
- 1 cup coconut water
- 1/2 cup ice cubes

Optional Additions:

- 1 teaspoon spirulina powder
- 1 tablespoon hemp seeds
- 1 tablespoon honey or maple syrup (for sweetness)

Directions:

1. In a blender, combine spinach, kale, mango chunks, avocado, chia seeds, coconut water, and ice cubes.
2. Blend until smooth and creamy.
3. If desired, add optional additions such as spirulina powder, hemp seeds, or sweetener, and blend again until well combined.
4. Pour into glasses and serve immediately.

Nutrition Facts (per serving):

- Calories: 180
- Protein: 6g
- Carbohydrates: 20g
- Fat: 10g
- Fiber: 10g

Golden Turmeric Latte

- **Prep Time:** 5 mins

  Total Time: 10 mins

  Servings: 2 cups

Ingredients:

- 2 cups unsweetened almond milk
- 1 teaspoon ground turmeric
- 1/2 teaspoon ground cinnamon
- 1/4 teaspoon ground ginger

- Pinch of black pepper
- 1 tablespoon honey or maple syrup (optional)
- Coconut oil (optional, for added healthy fats)

Directions:

1. In a small saucepan, heat almond milk over medium-low heat until warm but not boiling.
2. Whisk in ground turmeric, cinnamon, ginger, and black pepper until well combined.
3. If desired, add honey or maple syrup for sweetness, and coconut oil for added healthy fats.
4. Continue to heat, stirring frequently, until the latte is hot and well combined.
5. Pour into cups and serve immediately.

Nutrition Facts (per serving):

- Calories: 60
- Protein: 1g
- Carbohydrates: 9g
- Fat: 2g
- Fiber: 1g

Berry Blast Smoothie

- **Prep Time:** 5 mins

  Total Time: 5 mins

  Servings: 2 glasses

Ingredients:

- 1 cup frozen mixed berries
- 1 ripe banana

- 1/2 cup unsweetened almond milk
- 1 tablespoon chia seeds
- 1/2 cup ice cubes

Optional Toppings:

- Fresh berries
- Chopped nuts
- Unsweetened shredded coconut
- Granola

Directions:

1. In a blender, combine frozen mixed berries, banana, almond milk, chia seeds, and ice cubes.
2. Blend until smooth and creamy.
3. Pour into glasses and serve immediately.
4. If desired, top with fresh berries, chopped nuts, shredded coconut, or granola for added texture and flavor.

Nutrition Facts (per serving):

- Calories: 150
- Protein: 4g
- Carbohydrates: 25g
- Fat: 5g
- Fiber: 8g

DESSERTS RECIPES

Avocado Chocolate Mousse

- **Prep Time:** 10 mins

  Total Time: 10 mins

  Servings: 2

Ingredients:

- 1 ripe avocado
- 2 tablespoons unsweetened cocoa powder
- 2 tablespoons honey or maple syrup
- 1/2 teaspoon vanilla extract
- Pinch of salt
- Optional toppings: sliced strawberries, chopped nuts, coconut flakes

Directions:

1. Cut the avocado in half, remove the pit, and scoop the flesh into a blender or food processor.
2. Add cocoa powder, honey or maple syrup, vanilla extract, and a pinch of salt to the blender.
3. Blend until smooth and creamy, scraping down the sides of the blender as needed.
4. Divide the mousse into serving glasses or bowls.
5. Refrigerate for at least 30 minutes before serving.
6. Garnish with sliced strawberries, chopped nuts, or coconut flakes if desired.

Nutrition Facts (per serving):

- Calories: 190
- Protein: 3g
- Carbohydrates: 23g
- Fat: 12g
- Fiber: 8g

Chia Seed Pudding

- **Prep Time:** 5 mins

  Total Time: 4 hours (chilling time)

  Servings: 2

Ingredients:

- 1/4 cup chia seeds
- 1 cup unsweetened almond milk
- 1 tablespoon honey or maple syrup
- 1/2 teaspoon vanilla extract
- Optional toppings: fresh berries, sliced banana, nuts, shredded coconut

Directions:

1. In a bowl, combine chia seeds, almond milk, honey or maple syrup, and vanilla extract.
2. Stir well to combine.
3. Cover the bowl and refrigerate for at least 4 hours or overnight, stirring occasionally to prevent clumping.
4. Once the pudding has thickened to your desired consistency, divide it into serving glasses or bowls.
5. Top with fresh berries, sliced banana, nuts, or shredded coconut before serving.

Nutrition Facts (per serving):

- Calories: 150
- Protein: 4g
- Carbohydrates: 20g
- Fat: 7g
- Fiber: 10g

Coconut Mango Popsicles

- **Prep Time:** 10 mins

  Total Time: 4 hours (freezing time)

  Servings: 4 popsicles

Ingredients:

- 1 cup diced ripe mango
- 1/2 cup coconut milk
- 1 tablespoon honey or maple syrup
- 1/2 teaspoon vanilla extract

Directions:

1. In a blender, combine diced mango, coconut milk, honey or maple syrup, and vanilla extract.
2. Blend until smooth and creamy.
3. Pour the mixture into popsicle molds.
4. Insert popsicle sticks into each mold.
5. Freeze for at least 4 hours or until solid.
6. To remove the popsicles from the molds, run warm water over the outside of the molds for a few seconds.

Nutrition Facts (per serving):

- Calories: 90

- Protein: 1g
- Carbohydrates: 15g
- Fat: 4g
- Fiber: 1g

Greek Yogurt Parfait

- **Prep Time:** 5 mins
  Total Time: 5 mins
  Servings: 2

Ingredients:

- 1 cup Greek yogurt
- 1/2 cup mixed berries (such as strawberries, blueberries, raspberries)
- 2 tablespoons granola
- 1 tablespoon honey or maple syrup (optional)

Directions:

1. In serving glasses or bowls, layer Greek yogurt, mixed berries, and granola.
2. If desired, drizzle honey or maple syrup over the top for added sweetness.
3. Serve immediately.

Nutrition Facts (per serving):

- Calories: 160
- Protein: 12g
- Carbohydrates: 20g
- Fat: 4g
- Fiber: 3g

Banana Ice Cream

- **Prep Time:** 5 mins

  Total Time: 2 hours (freezing time)

  Servings: 2

Ingredients:

- 2 ripe bananas, peeled and sliced
- 1 tablespoon unsweetened cocoa powder (optional)
- 1 tablespoon peanut butter (optional)
- Optional toppings: sliced banana, chopped nuts, dark chocolate chips

Directions:

1. Place sliced bananas on a baking sheet lined with parchment paper.
2. Freeze for at least 2 hours or until firm.
3. Once frozen, transfer the bananas to a blender or food processor.
4. Add cocoa powder and peanut butter if desired.
5. Blend until smooth and creamy, scraping down the sides of the blender as needed.
6. Divide the banana ice cream into serving bowls.
7. Top with sliced banana, chopped nuts, or dark chocolate chips if desired.

Nutrition Facts (per serving without toppings):

- Calories: 100
- Protein: 1g
- Carbohydrates: 25g

- Fat: 0g
- Fiber: 3g

Raw Chocolate Energy Balls

- **Prep Time:** 15 mins

  Total Time: 15 mins

  Servings: 12 balls

Ingredients:

- 1 cup rolled oats
- 1/2 cup almond butter
- 1/4 cup raw honey or maple syrup
- 1/4 cup unsweetened cocoa powder
- 1 teaspoon vanilla extract
- Pinch of salt
- 1/4 cup chopped nuts (such as almonds, walnuts, or pecans)
- Optional: shredded coconut, chia seeds, or hemp seeds for coating

Directions:

1. In a food processor, combine rolled oats, almond butter, honey or maple syrup, cocoa powder, vanilla extract, and a pinch of salt.
2. Pulse until the mixture comes together and forms a dough-like consistency.
3. Add chopped nuts and pulse a few more times until the nuts are incorporated into the mixture.
4. Roll the mixture into small balls, about 1 inch in diameter.

5. If desired, roll the balls in shredded coconut, chia seeds, or hemp seeds for coating.

6. Place the energy balls on a plate or baking sheet lined with parchment paper.

7. Refrigerate for at least 30 minutes before serving.

Nutrition Facts (per ball):

- Calories: 120
- Protein: 3g
- Carbohydrates: 12g
- Fat: 7g
- Fiber: 2g

Frozen Yogurt Bark

- **Prep Time:** 10 mins

  Total Time: 2 hours (freezing time)

  Servings: 8 servings

Ingredients:

- 2 cups Greek yogurt
- 1 tablespoon honey or maple syrup
- 1/2 teaspoon vanilla extract
- 1/4 cup mixed berries (such as strawberries, blueberries, raspberries)
- 2 tablespoons chopped nuts (such as almonds or walnuts)
- Optional: dark chocolate chips, shredded coconut

Directions:

1. In a bowl, mix Greek yogurt, honey or maple syrup, and vanilla extract until well combined.

2. Line a baking sheet with parchment paper.

3. Spread the yogurt mixture evenly onto the parchment paper, about 1/4 inch thick.

4. Sprinkle mixed berries, chopped nuts, and any optional toppings evenly over the yogurt.

5. Place the baking sheet in the freezer and freeze for at least 2 hours or until firm.

6. Once frozen, break the yogurt bark into pieces and serve immediately.

Nutrition Facts (per serving):

- Calories: 70
- Protein: 5g
- Carbohydrates: 7g
- Fat: 3g
- Fiber: 1g

Baked Apple Slices

- **Prep Time:** 10 mins
  Total Time: 30 mins
  Servings: 2 servings

Ingredients:

- 1 large apple, cored and thinly sliced
- 1 tablespoon melted coconut oil
- 1 tablespoon honey or maple syrup
- 1/2 teaspoon ground cinnamon
- Pinch of nutmeg
- Pinch of salt

Directions:

1. Preheat the oven to 350°F (175°C).
2. In a bowl, toss apple slices with melted coconut oil, honey or maple syrup, ground cinnamon, nutmeg, and a pinch of salt until well coated.
3. Arrange the apple slices in a single layer on a baking sheet lined with parchment paper.
4. Bake for 20-25 minutes or until the apples are tender and lightly golden brown.
5. Serve warm as is or with a dollop of Greek yogurt on top.

Nutrition Facts (per serving):

- Calories: 120
- Protein: 0g
- Carbohydrates: 20g
- Fat: 5g
- Fiber: 3g

Frozen Banana Bites

- **Prep Time:** 10 mins

  Total Time: 2 hours (freezing time)

  Servings: 4 servings

Ingredients:

- 2 ripe bananas, peeled and cut into chunks
- 1/4 cup almond butter
- 1/4 cup dark chocolate chips
- 2 tablespoons chopped nuts (such as almonds or walnuts)
- Optional: shredded coconut, chia seeds

Directions:

1. Line a baking sheet with parchment paper.
2. Spread almond butter onto banana chunks and sandwich them together to form banana bites.
3. Place the banana bites on the prepared baking sheet.
4. Melt dark chocolate chips in the microwave or over a double boiler until smooth.
5. Drizzle melted chocolate over the banana bites.
6. Sprinkle chopped nuts and any optional toppings over the chocolate.
7. Place the baking sheet in the freezer and freeze for at least 2 hours or until the chocolate is set.
8. Serve chilled.

Nutrition Facts (per serving):

- Calories: 180
- Protein: 4g
- Carbohydrates: 22g
- Fat: 10g
- Fiber: 3g

Chocolate Avocado Pudding

- **Prep Time:** 10 mins

  Total Time: 10 mins

  Servings: 2

Ingredients:

- 1 ripe avocado
- 2 tablespoons unsweetened cocoa powder

- 2 tablespoons honey or maple syrup
- 1/2 teaspoon vanilla extract
- Pinch of salt
- Optional toppings: sliced strawberries, chopped nuts, shredded coconut

Directions:

1. Scoop out the flesh of the avocado and place it in a blender or food processor.
2. Add cocoa powder, honey or maple syrup, vanilla extract, and a pinch of salt.
3. Blend until smooth and creamy, scraping down the sides as needed.
4. Transfer the pudding into serving glasses or bowls.
5. Refrigerate for at least 30 minutes before serving.
6. Garnish with sliced strawberries, chopped nuts, or shredded coconut if desired.

Nutrition Facts (per serving):

- Calories: 190
- Protein: 3g
- Carbohydrates: 23g
- Fat: 12g
- Fiber: 8g

Chia Seed Chocolate Pudding

- **Prep Time:** 5 mins

  Total Time: 4 hours (chilling time)

  Servings: 2

Ingredients:

- 1/4 cup chia seeds
- 1 cup unsweetened almond milk
- 2 tablespoons cocoa powder
- 1 tablespoon honey or maple syrup
- 1/2 teaspoon vanilla extract
- Optional toppings: sliced banana, raspberries, shaved dark chocolate

Directions:

1. In a bowl, whisk together chia seeds, almond milk, cocoa powder, honey or maple syrup, and vanilla extract.
2. Mix well to combine all ingredients thoroughly.
3. Cover the bowl and refrigerate for at least 4 hours or overnight, stirring occasionally.
4. Once the pudding is set and thickened, divide it into serving bowls or glasses.
5. Garnish with sliced banana, raspberries, or shaved dark chocolate before serving.

Nutrition Facts (per serving):

- Calories: 160
- Protein: 5g
- Carbohydrates: 20g
- Fat: 8g
- Fiber: 10g

Berry Frozen Yogurt

- **Prep Time:** 5 mins

  Total Time: 4 hours (freezing time)

  Servings: 2

Ingredients:

- 1 cup frozen mixed berries
- 1/2 cup plain Greek yogurt
- 2 tablespoons honey or maple syrup
- 1 teaspoon lemon juice

Directions:

1. In a blender or food processor, combine frozen berries, Greek yogurt, honey or maple syrup, and lemon juice.
2. Blend until smooth and creamy.
3. Transfer the mixture into a shallow dish and spread it evenly.
4. Place the dish in the freezer for at least 4 hours or until firm.
5. Before serving, let the frozen yogurt sit at room temperature for a few minutes to soften slightly.
6. Scoop into serving bowls and enjoy!

Nutrition Facts (per serving):

- Calories: 120
- Protein: 6g
- Carbohydrates: 25g
- Fat: 1g
- Fiber: 5g

Coconut Almond Energy Balls

- **Prep Time:** 10 mins

  Total Time: 10 mins

  Servings: 8 balls

Ingredients:

- 1/2 cup rolled oats
- 1/4 cup almond butter
- 2 tablespoons honey or maple syrup
- 2 tablespoons shredded coconut
- 2 tablespoons chopped almonds
- 1/2 teaspoon vanilla extract
- Pinch of salt

Directions:

1. In a mixing bowl, combine rolled oats, almond butter, honey or maple syrup, shredded coconut, chopped almonds, vanilla extract, and a pinch of salt.
2. Mix until well combined and the mixture holds together.
3. Roll the mixture into small balls using your hands.
4. Place the energy balls on a plate or baking sheet lined with parchment paper.
5. Refrigerate for at least 30 minutes before serving.
6. Store any leftovers in an airtight container in the refrigerator.

Nutrition Facts (per serving - 1 ball):

- Calories: 90
- Protein: 3g
- Carbohydrates: 10g
- Fat: 5g

- Fiber: 2g

Berry Greek Yogurt Parfait

- **Prep Time:** 10 mins
- **Total Time:** 10 mins
- **Servings:** 2

Ingredients:

- 1 cup plain Greek yogurt
- 1 cup mixed berries (blueberries, raspberries, strawberries)
- 1/4 cup granola
- 1 tablespoon honey or maple syrup (optional)

Directions:

1. In two glasses, layer Greek yogurt, mixed berries, and granola alternately.
2. Repeat the layering process until glasses are full.
3. Drizzle honey or maple syrup over the top if desired.
4. Serve immediately as a refreshing dessert.

Nutritional Information (per serving):

- Calories: 200
- Protein: 15g
- Carbohydrates: 30g
- Fat: 3g
- Fiber: 6g

Coconut Chia Pudding

- **Prep Time:** 5 mins (+4 hours chilling time)
- **Total Time:** 4 hours 5 mins

- **Servings:** 2

Ingredients:

- 1/4 cup chia seeds
- 1 cup unsweetened coconut milk
- 1 tablespoon honey or maple syrup
- 1/2 teaspoon vanilla extract
- Unsweetened shredded coconut, for garnish
- Fresh berries, for garnish

Directions:

1. In a bowl, mix chia seeds, coconut milk, honey or maple syrup, and vanilla extract.
2. Cover and refrigerate for at least 4 hours or overnight, stirring occasionally.
3. Once thickened, spoon the pudding into serving glasses.
4. Garnish with shredded coconut and fresh berries.
5. Serve chilled.

Nutritional Information (per serving):

- Calories: 180
- Protein: 5g
- Carbohydrates: 15g
- Fat: 12g
- Fiber: 8g

Almond Butter Banana Bites

- **Prep Time:** 10 mins
- **Total Time:** 10 mins
- **Servings:** 2

Ingredients:

- 1 large ripe banana, sliced
- 2 tablespoons almond butter
- 2 tablespoons granola
- 1 tablespoon dark chocolate chips (optional)

Directions:

1. Spread almond butter on banana slices.
2. Press granola and chocolate chips onto the almond butter.
3. Serve immediately as a tasty and nutritious dessert.

Nutritional Information (per serving):

- Calories: 210
- Protein: 5g
- Carbohydrates: 30g
- Fat: 10g
- Fiber: 5g

Baked Apples with Cinnamon

- **Prep Time:** 10 mins
- **Total Time:** 40 mins
- **Servings:** 2

Ingredients:

- 2 apples, cored and halved
- 2 tablespoons honey or maple syrup
- 1/2 teaspoon ground cinnamon
- 1 tablespoon chopped nuts (walnuts or almonds)

Directions:

1. Preheat oven to 350°F (175°C).

2. Place apple halves in a baking dish, cut side up.

3. Drizzle honey or maple syrup over the apples.

4. Sprinkle with ground cinnamon and chopped nuts.

5. Bake for 30-35 minutes until apples are tender.

6. Serve warm, optionally with a dollop of Greek yogurt or a sprinkle of granola.

Nutritional Information (per serving):

- Calories: 150
- Protein: 2g
- Carbohydrates: 35g
- Fat: 3g
- Fiber: 6g

Chocolate Banana Ice Cream

- **Prep Time:** 5 mins (+4 hours freezing time)
- **Total Time:** 4 hours 5 mins
- **Servings:** 2

Ingredients:

- 2 ripe bananas, sliced and frozen
- 2 tablespoons cocoa powder
- 1 tablespoon honey or maple syrup
- 1/4 cup unsweetened almond milk
- 1/2 teaspoon vanilla extract

Directions:

1. In a blender, combine frozen banana slices, cocoa powder, honey or maple syrup, almond milk, and vanilla extract.

2. Blend until smooth and creamy, scraping down the sides as needed.

3. Transfer the mixture into a container and freeze for at least 4 hours.

4. Scoop into bowls and serve as a guilt-free chocolate dessert.

Nutritional Information (per serving):

- Calories: 160
- Protein: 2g
- Carbohydrates: 40g
- Fat: 1g
- Fiber: 5g

SALAD RECIPES

Quinoa and Kale Salad

- **Prep Time:** 10 mins
- **Total Time:** 20 mins
- **Servings:** 4

Ingredients:

- 1 cup quinoa, rinsed
- 2 cups water
- 4 cups kale, chopped
- 1 red bell pepper, diced
- 1 cucumber, diced
- 1/4 cup red onion, finely chopped
- 1/4 cup fresh parsley, chopped
- 1/4 cup feta cheese, crumbled (optional)
- 2 tablespoons olive oil
- 2 tablespoons lemon juice
- Salt and pepper to taste

Directions:

1. In a saucepan, bring quinoa and water to a boil. Reduce heat, cover, and simmer for 15 minutes, or until quinoa is cooked and water is absorbed. Remove from heat and let it cool.

2. In a large bowl, combine cooked quinoa, chopped kale, bell pepper, cucumber, red onion, and parsley.

3. In a small bowl, whisk together olive oil, lemon juice, salt, and pepper. Pour the dressing over the salad and toss to combine.

4. Top with crumbled feta cheese if desired.

5. Serve chilled or at room temperature.

Nutritional Information (per serving):

- Calories: 250

- Protein: 9g

- Carbohydrates: 32g

- Fat: 10g

- Fiber: 5g

Strawberry Spinach Salad

- **Prep Time:** 10 mins

- **Total Time:** 10 mins

- **Servings:** 4

Ingredients:

- 6 cups baby spinach

- 1 cup strawberries, sliced

- 1/4 cup red onion, thinly sliced

- 1/4 cup feta cheese, crumbled

- 1/4 cup sliced almonds

- 2 tablespoons balsamic vinegar

- 1 tablespoon olive oil

- 1 teaspoon honey

- Salt and pepper to taste

Directions:

1. In a large bowl, combine baby spinach, sliced strawberries, red onion, feta cheese, and sliced almonds.

2. In a small bowl, whisk together balsamic vinegar, olive oil, honey, salt, and pepper to make the dressing.

3. Pour the dressing over the salad and toss to coat evenly.

4. Serve immediately as a refreshing and nutritious salad option.

Nutritional Information (per serving):

- Calories: 150

- Protein: 5g

- Carbohydrates: 10g

- Fat: 10g

- Fiber: 4g

Mediterranean Chickpea Salad

- **Prep Time:** 10 mins

- **Total Time:** 10 mins

- **Servings:** 4

Ingredients:

- 1 can (15 oz.) chickpeas, drained and rinsed

- 1 cup cherry tomatoes, halved

- 1/2 English cucumber, diced

- 1/4 cup Kalamata olives, sliced

- 1/4 cup red onion, finely chopped

- 1/4 cup fresh parsley, chopped

- 2 tablespoons extra virgin olive oil

- 1 tablespoon lemon juice

- 1 teaspoon dried oregano

- Salt and pepper to taste

- Crumbled feta cheese (optional)

Directions:

1. In a large bowl, combine chickpeas, cherry tomatoes, cucumber, olives, red onion, and parsley.
2. In a small bowl, whisk together olive oil, lemon juice, dried oregano, salt, and pepper to make the dressing.
3. Pour the dressing over the salad and toss to combine.
4. Top with crumbled feta cheese if desired.
5. Serve immediately as a satisfying and flavorful salad.

Nutritional Information (per serving):

- Calories: 220
- Protein: 7g
- Carbohydrates: 25g
- Fat: 10g
- Fiber: 6g

Asian Quinoa Salad

- **Prep Time:** 15 mins
- **Total Time:** 20 mins
- **Servings:** 4

Ingredients:

- 1 cup quinoa, rinsed
- 2 cups water
- 1 red bell pepper, diced
- 1 cup shredded carrots
- 1 cup edamame, cooked
- 1/4 cup green onions, chopped
- 1/4 cup cilantro, chopped

- 2 tablespoons sesame seeds
- 1/4 cup soy sauce
- 2 tablespoons rice vinegar
- 1 tablespoon sesame oil
- 1 tablespoon honey
- 1 teaspoon grated ginger
- Salt and pepper to taste

Directions:

1. In a saucepan, bring quinoa and water to a boil. Reduce heat, cover, and simmer for 15 minutes, or until quinoa is cooked and water is absorbed. Remove from heat and let it cool.

2. In a large bowl, combine cooked quinoa, diced bell pepper, shredded carrots, edamame, green onions, cilantro, and sesame seeds.

3. In a small bowl, whisk together soy sauce, rice vinegar, sesame oil, honey, grated ginger, salt, and pepper to make the dressing.

4. Pour the dressing over the salad and toss to coat evenly.

5. Serve chilled or at room temperature.

Nutritional Information (per serving):

- Calories: 280
- Protein: 10g
- Carbohydrates: 35g
- Fat: 10g
- Fiber: 7g

Avocado and Tomato Salad

- **Prep Time:** 10 mins

- **Total Time:** 10 mins
- **Servings:** 2

Ingredients:

- 1 ripe avocado, diced
- 1 cup cherry tomatoes, halved
- 1/4 cup red onion, finely chopped
- 2 tablespoons fresh parsley, chopped
- 1 tablespoon extra-virgin olive oil
- 1 tablespoon balsamic vinegar
- Salt and pepper to taste

Directions:

1. In a salad bowl, combine diced avocado, halved cherry tomatoes, chopped red onion, and fresh parsley.
2. Drizzle with olive oil and balsamic vinegar.
3. Season with salt and pepper according to taste.
4. Gently toss the ingredients until evenly coated.
5. Serve immediately as a refreshing and nutritious salad option.

Nutritional Information (per serving):

- Calories: 180
- Protein: 2g
- Carbohydrates: 10g
- Fat: 15g
- Fiber: 6g

Quinoa and Black Bean Salad

- **Prep Time:** 15 mins
- **Total Time:** 25 mins

- **Servings:** 4

Ingredients:

- 1 cup quinoa, rinsed
- 2 cups water
- 1 can (15 oz) black beans, drained and rinsed
- 1 cup corn kernels
- 1 red bell pepper, diced
- 1/4 cup red onion, finely chopped
- 1/4 cup fresh cilantro, chopped
- 2 tablespoons lime juice
- 2 tablespoons olive oil
- 1 teaspoon ground cumin
- Salt and pepper to taste

Directions:

1. In a saucepan, bring quinoa and water to a boil. Reduce heat, cover, and simmer for 15 minutes, or until quinoa is cooked and water is absorbed. Remove from heat and let it cool.
2. In a large bowl, combine cooked quinoa, black beans, corn kernels, diced bell pepper, chopped red onion, and chopped cilantro.
3. In a small bowl, whisk together lime juice, olive oil, ground cumin, salt, and pepper to make the dressing.
4. Pour the dressing over the salad and toss to combine.
5. Serve chilled or at room temperature.

Nutritional Information (per serving):

- Calories: 320

- Protein: 11g
- Carbohydrates: 48g
- Fat: 9g
- Fiber: 10g

Spinach and Strawberry Salad

- **Prep Time:** 10 mins
- **Total Time:** 10 mins
- **Servings:** 2

Ingredients:

- 4 cups baby spinach
- 1 cup strawberries, sliced
- 1/4 cup almonds, sliced
- 2 tablespoons balsamic vinegar
- 1 tablespoon honey
- 1 tablespoon extra-virgin olive oil
- Salt and pepper to taste

Directions:

1. In a large bowl, combine baby spinach, sliced strawberries, and sliced almonds.
2. In a small bowl, whisk together balsamic vinegar, honey, olive oil, salt, and pepper to make the dressing.
3. Pour the dressing over the salad and toss to coat evenly.
4. Serve immediately as a delightful and nutritious salad option.

Nutritional Information (per serving):

- Calories: 210
- Protein: 5g

- Carbohydrates: 22g
- Fat: 13g
- Fiber: 6g

Greek Salad

- **Prep Time:** 15 mins
- **Total Time:** 15 mins
- **Servings:** 4

Ingredients:

- 2 cups cucumber, diced
- 2 cups cherry tomatoes, halved
- 1/2 cup red onion, thinly sliced
- 1/4 cup Kalamata olives, sliced
- 1/4 cup crumbled feta cheese
- 2 tablespoons extra virgin olive oil
- 1 tablespoon red wine vinegar
- 1 teaspoon dried oregano
- Salt and pepper to taste

Directions:

1. In a large bowl, combine diced cucumber, halved cherry tomatoes, thinly sliced red onion, sliced Kalamata olives, and crumbled feta cheese.
2. In a small bowl, whisk together olive oil, red wine vinegar, dried oregano, salt, and pepper to make the dressing.
3. Pour the dressing over the salad and toss to coat evenly.
4. Serve immediately as a delicious and satisfying salad.

Nutritional Information (per serving):

- Calories: 170
- Protein: 5g
- Carbohydrates: 10g
- Fat: 14g
- Fiber: 3g

Asian Cabbage Salad

- **Prep Time:** 15 mins
- **Total Time:** 15 mins
- **Servings:** 4

Ingredients:

- 4 cups shredded cabbage
- 1 cup shredded carrots
- 1/4 cup sliced almonds
- 2 tablespoons chopped cilantro
- 2 tablespoons sesame seeds
- 2 tablespoons rice vinegar
- 1 tablespoon soy sauce
- 1 tablespoon honey
- 1 tablespoon sesame oil
- 1 teaspoon grated ginger
- Salt and pepper to taste

Directions:

1. In a large bowl, combine shredded cabbage, shredded carrots, sliced almonds, chopped cilantro, and sesame seeds.

2. In a small bowl, whisk together rice vinegar, soy sauce, honey, sesame oil, grated ginger, salt, and pepper to make the dressing.

3. Pour the dressing over the salad and toss to coat evenly.

4. Serve immediately as a flavorful and nutritious salad option.

Nutritional Information (per serving):

- Calories: 160

- Protein: 4g

- Carbohydrates: 20g

- Fat: 8g

- Fiber: 5g

Quinoa and Kale Salad

- **Prep Time:** 15 mins

- **Total Time:** 20 mins

- **Servings:** 4

Ingredients:

- 1 cup quinoa

- 2 cups water or vegetable broth

- 2 cups kale, chopped

- 1 cup cherry tomatoes, halved

- 1/4 cup red onion, thinly sliced

- 1/4 cup almonds, sliced

- 2 tablespoons olive oil

- 2 tablespoons lemon juice

- 1 teaspoon Dijon mustard

- Salt and pepper to taste

Directions:

- Rinse quinoa under cold water. In a saucepan, bring quinoa and water to a boil. Reduce heat, cover, and simmer for 15 minutes, or until quinoa is cooked and liquid is absorbed. Remove from heat and let it cool.

- In a large bowl, combine cooked quinoa, chopped kale, halved cherry tomatoes, thinly sliced red onion, and sliced almonds.
- In a small bowl, whisk together olive oil, lemon juice, Dijon mustard, salt, and pepper to make the dressing.
- Pour the dressing over the salad and toss to coat evenly.
- Serve immediately or refrigerate until ready to serve.

Nutritional Information (per serving):

- Calories: 270
- Protein: 9g
- Carbohydrates: 33g
- Fat: 12g
- Fiber: 6g

Beet and Goat Cheese Salad

- **Prep Time:** 10 mins
- **Total Time:** 30 mins
- **Servings:** 4
- **Ingredients:**
- 4 medium beets, roasted, peeled, and sliced
- 4 cups mixed greens (spinach, arugula, or mesclun)
- 1/4 cup walnuts, chopped
- 2 ounces' goat cheese, crumbled
- 2 tablespoons balsamic vinegar
- 1 tablespoon extra-virgin olive oil
- 1 teaspoon honey

- Salt and pepper to taste

Directions:

- Preheat the oven to 400°F (200°C). Wrap beets in aluminum foil and roast for about 45 minutes, or until tender. Let them cool, then peel and slice.
- In a large bowl, combine mixed greens, roasted beet slices, chopped walnuts, and crumbled goat cheese.
- In a small bowl, whisk together balsamic vinegar, olive oil, honey, salt, and pepper to make the dressing.
- Drizzle the dressing over the salad and toss gently to coat.
- Serve immediately for a delightful and colorful salad.

Nutritional Information (per serving):

- Calories: 220
- Protein: 7g
- Carbohydrates: 17g
- Fat: 14g
- Fiber: 4g

Mango and Avocado Salad

- **Prep Time:** 15 mins
- **Total Time:** 15 mins
- **Servings:** 4

Ingredients:

- 2 ripe mangoes, peeled and diced
- 2 ripe avocados, peeled and diced
- 1 cup cucumber, diced
- 1/4 cup red onion, thinly sliced

- 1/4 cup fresh cilantro, chopped
- 2 tablespoons lime juice
- 1 tablespoon olive oil
- Salt and pepper to taste

Directions:

- In a large bowl, combine diced mangoes, diced avocados, diced cucumber, thinly sliced red onion, and chopped cilantro.
- Drizzle lime juice and olive oil over the salad.
- Season with salt and pepper according to taste.
- Gently toss the ingredients until well combined.
- Serve immediately as a refreshing and nutritious salad option.

Nutritional Information (per serving):

- Calories: 220
- Protein: 3g
- Carbohydrates: 23g
- Fat: 15g
- Fiber: 8g

Greek Chickpea Salad

- **Prep Time:** 15 mins
- **Total Time:** 15 mins
- **Servings:** 4

Ingredients:

- 2 cups cooked chickpeas (canned or cooked from dry)
- 1 cup cucumber, diced
- 1 cup cherry tomatoes, halved
- 1/4 cup red onion, thinly sliced

- 1/4 cup Kalamata olives, sliced
- 1/4 cup crumbled feta cheese
- 2 tablespoons fresh parsley, chopped
- 2 tablespoons lemon juice
- 2 tablespoons extra virgin olive oil
- 1 teaspoon dried oregano
- Salt and pepper to taste

Directions:

- In a large bowl, combine cooked chickpeas, diced cucumber, halved cherry tomatoes, thinly sliced red onion, sliced Kalamata olives, crumbled feta cheese, and chopped parsley.
- In a small bowl, whisk together lemon juice, olive oil, dried oregano, salt, and pepper to make the dressing.
- Pour the dressing over the salad and toss to coat evenly.
- Serve immediately or refrigerate until ready to serve.

Nutritional Information (per serving):

- Calories: 270
- Protein: 10g
- Carbohydrates: 28g
- Fat: 13g
- Fiber: 8g

Quinoa Avocado Salad

- **Prep Time:** 10 mins
- **Total Time:** 25 mins
- **Servings:** 4

Ingredients:

- 1 cup quinoa, rinsed
- 2 cups water or vegetable broth
- 1 avocado, diced
- 1 cup cherry tomatoes, halved
- 1/4 cup red onion, finely chopped
- 1/4 cup fresh cilantro, chopped
- 2 tablespoons lime juice
- 2 tablespoons olive oil
- Salt and pepper to taste

Directions:

1. In a saucepan, bring water or vegetable broth to a boil. Add quinoa, cover, and simmer for 15-20 minutes until quinoa is cooked and water is absorbed. Remove from heat and let it cool.

2. In a large bowl, combine cooked quinoa, diced avocado, halved cherry tomatoes, chopped red onion, and chopped cilantro.

3. In a small bowl, whisk together lime juice, olive oil, salt, and pepper to make the dressing.

4. Pour the dressing over the salad and toss gently to coat.

5. Serve immediately or chill in the refrigerator for 30 minutes before serving.

Nutritional Information (per serving):

- Calories: 280
- Protein: 7g
- Carbohydrates: 30g
- Fat: 15g
- Fiber: 6g

Greek Salad with Chickpeas

- **Prep Time:** 15 mins
- **Total Time:** 15 mins
- **Servings:** 4

Ingredients:

- 2 cups mixed greens (romaine, spinach, arugula)
- 1 cup cherry tomatoes, halved
- 1 cucumber, diced
- 1/4 cup red onion, thinly sliced
- 1/4 cup Kalamata olives, sliced
- 1/4 cup crumbled feta cheese
- 1 cup cooked chickpeas (canned or boiled)
- 2 tablespoons extra virgin olive oil
- 2 tablespoons red wine vinegar
- 1 teaspoon dried oregano
- Salt and pepper to taste

Directions:

1. In a large bowl, combine mixed greens, halved cherry tomatoes, diced cucumber, thinly sliced red onion, sliced Kalamata olives, crumbled feta cheese, and cooked chickpeas.
2. In a small bowl, whisk together olive oil, red wine vinegar, dried oregano, salt, and pepper to make the dressing.
3. Pour the dressing over the salad and toss to coat evenly.
4. Serve immediately as a refreshing and nutritious meal.

Nutritional Information (per serving):

- Calories: 280

- Protein: 9g

- Carbohydrates: 22g

- Fat: 17g

- Fiber: 7g

Spinach Strawberry Salad

- **Prep Time:** 10 mins

- **Total Time:** 10 mins

- **Servings:** 4

Ingredients:

- 4 cups baby spinach

- 1 cup strawberries, sliced

- 1/4 cup sliced almonds

- 1/4 cup feta cheese, crumbled

- 2 tablespoons balsamic vinegar

- 1 tablespoon honey

- 1 tablespoon olive oil

- Salt and pepper to taste

Directions:

1. In a large bowl, combine baby spinach, sliced strawberries, sliced almonds, and crumbled feta cheese.

2. In a small bowl, whisk together balsamic vinegar, honey, olive oil, salt, and pepper to make the dressing.

3. Pour the dressing over the salad and toss gently to coat.

4. Serve immediately as a delightful and colorful salad option.

Nutritional Information (per serving):

- Calories: 180

- Protein: 5g

- Carbohydrates: 15g

- Fat: 11g

- Fiber: 4g

Asian Cabbage Salad

- **Prep Time:** 15 mins

- **Total Time:** 15 mins

- **Servings:** 4

Ingredients:

- 4 cups shredded cabbage (green or purple)

- 1 cup shredded carrots

- 1/4 cup sliced green onions

- 1/4 cup chopped cilantro

- 1/4 cup sliced almonds

- 2 tablespoons sesame seeds

- 2 tablespoons soy sauce

- 1 tablespoon rice vinegar

- 1 tablespoon sesame oil

- 1 tablespoon honey

- 1 teaspoon grated ginger

- 1 clove garlic, minced

Directions:

1. In a large bowl, combine shredded cabbage, shredded carrots, sliced green onions, chopped cilantro, sliced almonds, and sesame seeds.

2. In a small bowl, whisk together soy sauce, rice vinegar, sesame oil, honey, grated ginger, and minced garlic to make the dressing.

3. Pour the dressing over the salad and toss to coat evenly.

4. Serve immediately as a crunchy and flavorful salad option.

Nutritional Information (per serving):

- Calories: 180
- Protein: 6g
- Carbohydrates: 18g
- Fat: 10g
- Fiber: 5g

MEAL PLAN

Day 1

- **Breakfast:** Microbiome Smoothie
- **Lunch:** Quinoa Avocado Salad
- **Dinner:** Greek Salad with Chickpeas

Day 2

- **Breakfast:** Spinach Strawberry Salad
- **Lunch:** Mediterranean Chickpea Salad
- **Dinner:** Apple Walnut Salad

Day 3

- **Breakfast:** Microbiome Smoothie
- **Lunch:** Asian Cabbage Salad
- **Dinner:** Caprese Salad

Day 4

- **Breakfast:** Quinoa Avocado Salad
- **Lunch:** Thai Peanut Salad
- **Dinner:** Spinach and Quinoa Salad

Day 5

- **Breakfast:** Microbiome Smoothie
- **Lunch:** Mexican Corn Salad
- **Dinner:** Greek Salad with Chickpeas

Day 6

- **Breakfast:** Spinach Strawberry Salad

- **Lunch:** Apple Walnut Salad
- **Dinner:** Mediterranean Chickpea Salad

Day 7

- **Breakfast:** Microbiome Smoothie
- **Lunch:** Caprese Salad
- **Dinner:** Asian Cabbage Salad

Day 8

- **Breakfast:** Quinoa Avocado Salad
- **Lunch:** Thai Peanut Salad
- **Dinner:** Mexican Corn Salad

Day 9

- **Breakfast:** Microbiome Smoothie
- **Lunch:** Spinach and Quinoa Salad
- **Dinner:** Apple Walnut Salad

Day 10

- **Breakfast:** Spinach Strawberry Salad
- **Lunch:** Mediterranean Chickpea Salad
- **Dinner:** Greek Salad with Chickpeas

Day 11

- **Breakfast:** Microbiome Smoothie
- **Lunch:** Caprese Salad
- **Dinner:** Thai Peanut Salad

Day 12

- **Breakfast:** Quinoa Avocado Salad

- **Lunch:** Mexican Corn Salad

- **Dinner:** Asian Cabbage Salad

Day 13

- **Breakfast:** Microbiome Smoothie

- **Lunch:** Apple Walnut Salad

- **Dinner:** Spinach and Quinoa Salad

Day 14

- **Breakfast:** Mediterranean Chickpea Salad

- **Lunch:** Greek Salad with Chickpeas

- **Dinner:** Caprese Salad

Day 15

- **Breakfast:** Microbiome Smoothie

- **Lunch:** Thai Peanut Salad

- **Dinner:** Mexican Corn Salad

Day 16

- **Breakfast:** Quinoa Avocado Salad

- **Lunch:** Spinach Strawberry Salad

- **Dinner:** Asian Cabbage Salad

Day 17

- **Breakfast:** Microbiome Smoothie

- **Lunch:** Apple Walnut Salad

- **Dinner:** Caprese Salad

Day 18

- **Breakfast:** Greek Salad with Chickpeas
- **Lunch:** Mediterranean Chickpea Salad
- **Dinner:** Thai Peanut Salad

Day 19

- **Breakfast:** Microbiome Smoothie
- **Lunch:** Spinach and Quinoa Salad
- **Dinner:** Mexican Corn Salad

Day 20

- **Breakfast:** Quinoa Avocado Salad
- **Lunch:** Asian Cabbage Salad
- **Dinner:** Apple Walnut Salad

Day 21

- **Breakfast:** Microbiome Smoothie
- **Lunch:** Greek Salad with Chickpeas
- **Dinner:** Caprese Salad

TIPS FOR DINING OUT WITH THE METABOLIC CONFUSION DIET

In today's fast-paced world, dining out has become a common occurrence for many individuals. However, sticking to a specific diet plan, such as the metabolic confusion diet, can present challenges when faced with restaurant menus and social events. In this chapter, we will explore practical tips and strategies for making healthy choices at restaurants and navigating social events while adhering to the principles of the metabolic confusion diet.

Making Healthy Choices at Restaurants

Dining out can often tempt us with indulgent options that may not align with our dietary goals. However, with some preparation and mindful decision-making, it is possible to enjoy restaurant meals while staying true to the metabolic confusion diet.

One of the first steps in making healthy choices at restaurants is to research the menu beforehand, if possible. Many restaurants now offer online menus, allowing you to review the options and plan your meal in advance. Look for dishes that include lean protein, plenty of vegetables, and whole grains. Avoid items that are fried, heavily processed, or loaded with added sugars and unhealthy fats.

When ordering, don't be afraid to ask questions or request modifications to suit your dietary needs. Most restaurants are willing to accommodate special requests, such as substituting steamed vegetables for french fries or asking for dressing on the side. Additionally, consider splitting entrees with a dining companion or ordering appetizers as your main course to control portion sizes.

Another helpful tip is to be mindful of portion sizes. Restaurant servings are often much larger than what we would typically eat at home. Consider asking for a to-go box upfront and portioning out half of your meal to enjoy later. This not only helps with portion control but also allows you to enjoy your favorite dishes without overindulging.

Lastly, listen to your body's hunger and fullness cues. Eat slowly and savor each bite, paying attention to how your body feels throughout the meal. Stop eating when you feel satisfied, even if there is food left on your plate. Remember, it's okay to leave food behind if you are no longer hungry.

By following these tips, you can enjoy dining out while staying on track with your metabolic confusion diet goals.

Navigating Social Events with the Metabolic Confusion Diet

Social events and gatherings can present unique challenges for individuals following a specific diet plan. Whether it's a birthday party, wedding reception, or office luncheon, it's important to have strategies in place to navigate these situations while maintaining your dietary goals.

One of the most effective strategies for navigating social events is to plan ahead. If you know you'll be attending an event where food will be served, consider eating a small, balanced meal or snack beforehand to help curb hunger and prevent overeating. Additionally, bring along a healthy dish to share with others, ensuring that there will be at least one option available that aligns with your dietary preferences.

When faced with a buffet or potluck-style meal, take a lap around the table before filling your plate. This allows you to assess all the available options and make mindful choices about what to include on your plate. Look for lean protein sources, salads, and vegetables, and avoid loading up on high-calorie, low-nutrient items like chips, dips, and desserts.

Practice mindful eating during social events by paying attention to your body's hunger and fullness cues. Take small bites, chew slowly, and savor the flavors of each dish. Avoid mindlessly grazing or eating out of boredom, and focus on enjoying the company of those around you rather than solely on the food.

If alcohol is being served at the event, be mindful of your intake. Alcoholic beverages can be high in calories and may lower inhibitions, leading to overeating. Opt for light beer, wine spritzers, or mixed drinks made with low-calorie mixers, and alternate alcoholic beverages with water to stay hydrated.

Lastly, don't be too hard on yourself if you indulge in a treat or two during a social event. Remember that occasional indulgences are a normal part of life, and one off-plan meal or snack is unlikely to derail your progress. Focus on making healthy choices the majority of the time and practice self-compassion when deviations occur.

In conclusion, navigating social events while following the metabolic confusion diet requires planning, mindfulness, and flexibility. By implementing these strategies, you can enjoy social gatherings without compromising your dietary goals.

FREQUENTLY ASKED QUESTIONS

The metabolic confusion diet has gained popularity for its ability to boost metabolism, promote weight loss, and improve overall health. However, like any dietary approach, it also comes with its fair share of questions and concerns. In this chapter, we will address some of the most common inquiries about the metabolic confusion diet, as well as provide troubleshooting and adaptation tips for those embarking on this nutritional journey.

Common Concerns About the Metabolic Confusion Diet

- **Is the Metabolic Confusion Diet Safe?** The metabolic confusion diet is generally considered safe for healthiest individuals. However, as with any diet plan, it's essential to consult with a healthcare professional before making significant changes to your eating habits, especially if you have underlying health conditions or are pregnant or breastfeeding.

- **Will I Experience Side Effects?** Some individuals may experience mild side effects when first starting the metabolic confusion diet, such as headaches, fatigue, or digestive discomfort. These symptoms are typically temporary and often subside as the body adjusts to the new eating pattern. Staying hydrated, getting plenty of rest, and gradually introducing changes to your diet can help minimize side effects.

- **Can I Follow the Metabolic Confusion Diet Long-Term?** The metabolic confusion diet is designed to be followed in cycles, with periods of higher and lower calorie intake to prevent metabolic adaptation and promote fat loss. While some people may choose to incorporate elements of the diet into their long-term eating habits, it's essential to listen to your body's needs and make adjustments as necessary. Consulting with a registered dietitian can help you create a sustainable eating plan that aligns with your health goals.

- **Will I Lose Weight Quickly on the Metabolic Confusion Diet?** Weight loss results on the metabolic confusion diet can vary depending on individual factors such as starting weight, metabolism, activity level, and adherence to the program. Some people may experience rapid weight loss during the initial phases of the diet, while others may see more gradual progress over time. It's essential to focus on overall health and well-being rather than solely on the number on the scale.

Troubleshooting and Adaptation Tips

- **Plateauing on the Metabolic Confusion Diet** If you find yourself plateauing or experiencing a lack of progress on the metabolic confusion diet, consider reassessing your calorie intake and activity level. You may need to adjust your calorie cycling pattern or increase your exercise frequency or intensity to jumpstart weight loss. Additionally, incorporating more variety into your meals and snacks can help prevent boredom and keep your metabolism guessing.

- **Dealing with Hunger and Cravings** Hunger and cravings are common challenges when following any diet plan, including the metabolic confusion diet. To manage hunger, focus on including plenty of fiber-rich foods, lean protein sources, and healthy fats in your meals and snacks. Drinking water throughout the day can also help curb appetite and prevent overeating. If cravings strike, opt for nutritious alternatives such as fruit, nuts, or Greek yogurt to satisfy your sweet or savory tooth without derailing your progress.

- **Social Situations and Dining Out** Navigating social situations and dining out while following the metabolic confusion diet can be challenging but manageable with some planning and flexibility. Consider researching restaurant menus beforehand, making healthy choices, and practicing portion control. When attending social events, focus on enjoying the company of others rather than solely on the food, and remember that occasional indulgences are a normal part of life.

- **Listen to Your Body** Above all, listen to your body's hunger and fullness cues, and honor its needs. Pay attention to how different foods make you feel and adjust your eating patterns accordingly. Remember that the metabolic confusion diet is meant to be adaptable and flexible, allowing you to tailor it to your individual preferences and lifestyle.

CONCLUSION

In conclusion, the metabolic confusion diet offers a dynamic approach to weight loss and metabolic health by incorporating cycling patterns of calorie intake to prevent adaptation and optimize fat loss. Throughout this exploration, we've delved into various aspects of the diet, including its principles, benefits, meal plans, dining out tips, and troubleshooting strategies.

We've learned that the key to success with the metabolic confusion diet lies in its flexibility and adaptability. By cycling between periods of higher and lower calorie intake, individuals can keep their metabolism guessing, prevent plateaus, and achieve sustainable weight loss results. Additionally, incorporating nutrient-dense foods, staying hydrated, and engaging in regular physical activity are essential components of this dietary approach.

Moreover, we've discussed the importance of making healthy choices when dining out and navigating social events while following the metabolic confusion diet. With proper planning and mindfulness, individuals can enjoy meals outside of the home without compromising their health and wellness goals.

Furthermore, we addressed common concerns about the metabolic confusion diet, such as its safety, potential side effects, and long-term sustainability. By consulting with healthcare professionals, listening to their bodies, and making adjustments as needed, individuals can overcome challenges and achieve success with this dietary approach.

In essence, the metabolic confusion diet is not just about losing weight— it's about fostering a healthy relationship with food, optimizing metabolic health, and enhancing overall well-being. As we embark on our journey toward better health, let us remember the words of Hippocrates, the father of medicine, who famously said, "Let food be thy medicine and medicine be thy food." This timeless wisdom reminds us that the foods we eat have a profound impact on our health and vitality. So let us choose wisely, nourish our bodies with wholesome foods, and embrace the journey to a healthier, happier life.

9 798320 252285